Vulval Dermatologic Diagnosis

Vulval Dermatologic Diagnosis
Diagnosis by Clinical Presenting Sign

Giuseppe Micali, MD
Head of the Section of Dermatology and Venereology
University of Catania
Sicily, Italy

Pompeo Donofrio, MD
Dermatologist
Naples, Italy

Maria Rita Nasca, MD, PhD
Dermatology Clinic
University of Catania
Sicily, Italy

Stefano Veraldi, MD
Director of the School of Specialization in
Dermatology and Venereology
University of Milan
Milan, Italy

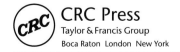

CRC Press
Taylor & Francis Group
Boca Raton London New York

CRC Press is an imprint of the
Taylor & Francis Group, an **informa** business

CRC Press
Taylor & Francis Group
6000 Broken Sound Parkway NW, Suite 300
Boca Raton, FL 33487-2742

© 2016 by Taylor & Francis Group, LLC
CRC Press is an imprint of Taylor & Francis Group, an Informa business

No claim to original U.S. Government works

Printed on acid-free paper
Version Date: 20150602

International Standard Book Number-13: 978-1-4822-2641-6 (Paperback)

Visit the Taylor & Francis Web site at
http://www.taylorandfrancis.com

and the CRC Press Web site at
http://www.crcpress.com

Contents

Editors

Professor Giuseppe Micali is head of the Department of Dermatology and director of the residency program in dermatology at the University of Catania, Italy. He graduated from, and then completed his residency training in dermatology and venereology at the University of Catania, Italy in 1986. Since then, he has served as a visiting faculty member on a number of occasions at the departments of dermatology at the University of Illinois, Northwestern University, and the University of Miami, USA. Professor Micali has actively participated as chairman and speaker at many national and international meetings, as well as in training courses related to dermatology. He has had longstanding scientific collaboration with several foreign universities, including the University of Illinois, Northwestern University, Rutgers-New Jersey Medical School and the University of Miami. He is also a member of various national and international societies, and a founding member of the Italian Board of Pediatric Dermatology, Italian Board of Research in Dermovenereologic Therapy, Italian Acne Board, Study Group on Cutaneous Appendages and the Mediterranean Acne Group. Professor Micali has authored over 400 publications, including 182 articles in peer-reviewed journals and 93 book chapters and he is editor of 16 books. He currently serves as an editorial board member of numerous international journals, including the *Journal of the American Academy of Dermatology* (USA), *Journal of Dermatologic Treatment* (USA), *International Journal of Dermatology* (USA), *Acta Dermatovenerologica Croatica*, and *European Journal of Acne*. In addition to having served on advisory boards for several pharmaceutical companies, Professor Micali is actively involved in clinical research of skin disorders. His main fields of interest include acne, dermatologic therapy, noninvasive diagnostic technologies, and genital disorders.

Professor Pompeo Donofrio is a specialist in dermatology and venereology. He was a senior researcher at the Dermatology Clinic of the University "Federico II," Naples, Italy from 1974 to 2009. Since then he has been medical director of the genital dermatology and sexually transmitted diseases (STDs) outpatient clinical service and faculty member at the residency program in dermatology and venereology at the Department of Dermatology of the University "Federico II," Naples, Italy. Since 1984 he has served as medical counselor for HIV patients at the Medical School Department of Communicable Diseases of the "Federico II" University, and at the Division of Infectious Diseases of "D. Cotugno" Hospital, Naples, Italy. He has actively been involved in university-based research programs sponsored by the Italian National Research Institute (CNR) and by the Italian Ministry of Scientific Research. He is author of over 200 scientific publications, including articles and book chapters. He has actively participated as chairman and speaker at many national and international meetings, as well as in training courses related to dermatology, STDs, and AIDS.

Doctor Maria Rita Nasca is a dermatologist member of the medical staff and teacher in the residency program in dermatology at the Dermatology Clinic of the University of Catania, Italy. She graduated from and then completed her residency training in dermatology and venereology at the University of Catania, Italy in 1994. She earned her PhD in dermatology, anatomy, and plastic surgery from the University "La Sapienza" of Rome, Italy in 2000. She was a visiting scholar in 1996, 1997, 1998, and 1999 at the Department of Dermatology of the Northwestern University, Chicago, Illinois, USA where she has carried out laboratory studies on the effects of thalidomide and of mechanical stress on epidermal keratinocytes, resulting in publications in high-quality peer-reviewed journals. She has authored over 140 publications, including book chapters and articles in national and international journals. Her main fields of interest and clinical research include HPV (human papillomavirus) infections, genital disorders, ectoparasitoses, autoimmune bullous disorders, lichen sclerosus, and other rare dermatologic diseases.

Professor Stefano Veraldi graduated in medicine and surgery from the University of Milan, Italy, in 1984. He was a research fellow at the Department of Dermatology, University of Milan, Italy, 1986–1988; specialist in dermatology and venereology, 1987; assistant dermatologist, 1990–2000; senior researcher, 2000–2002; associate professor, 2002–2014; and head of the Postgraduate School of Dermatology and Venereology at the University of Milan, 2013–2014. He was the cofounder of the Italian Group for the Study of Skin Ulcers (GISUC) in 1999; cofounder of the European Institute of Dermatology (Milan) in 2001, and cofounder of the Italian Acne Board (IAB) in 2004. Professor Veraldi was a visiting professor at the University of Uppsala, Sweden, 2004; scientific director of the European Institute of Dermatology, Milan, 2007–2008; president of the IAB 2009–2014; member of the Rosacea Global Advisory Board, 2012–2014; member of the European Severe Acne Board, 2014; and visiting professor at the University of Makallè, Ethiopia, 2014. He is the author of 26 books, 72 chapters in various books, 179 articles indexed on Scopus, 165 on Web of Science, and 138 on PubMed.

Contributors

Federica Dall'Oglio
Dermatology Clinic
University of Catania
Catania, Italy

Franco Dinotta
Dermatology Clinic
University of Catania
Catania, Italy

Paola Donofrio
School of Dermatology and Venereology
University of Naples "Federico II"
Naples, Italy

Pompeo Donofrio
School of Dermatology and Venereology
University of Naples "Federico II"
Naples, Italy

Giuseppe Giuffrida
Department of Gynecology
Lucina-Gretter Clinic
Catania, Italy

Francesco Lacarrubba
Dermatology Clinic
University of Catania
Catania, Italy

Ivano Luppino
Dermatology Clinic
University of Catania
Catania, Italy

Giuseppe Micali
Dermatology Clinic
University of Catania
Catania, Italy

Maria Letizia Musumeci
Dermatology Clinic
University of Catania
Catania, Italy

Maria Rita Nasca
Dermatology Clinic
University of Catania
Catania, Italy

Nella Pulvirenti
Dermatology Clinic
University of Catania
Catania, Italy

Aurora Tedeschi
Dermatology Clinic
University of Catania
Catania, Italy

Stefano Veraldi
Institute of Dermatological Sciences
University of Milan
IRCCS Foundation
Ospedale Maggiore Policlinico, Mangiagalli e
    Regina Elena
Milan, Italy

Anna Elisa Verzì
Dermatology Clinic
University of Catania
Catania, Italy

Introduction and Terminology

Vulvar disorders span through many aspects of gender medicine, including sexually transmitted infections and neoplastic disorders.

Professors Giuseppe Micali (Catania), Pompeo Donofrio (Naples), Maria Rita Nasca (Catania), and Stefano Veraldi (Milan) have consolidated experience in the diagnosis and management of genital disorders, confirmed by previous publications in this field, also including an *Atlas of Male Genital Disorders*. All four distinguished physician-scientists have worked on genital disorders for many years. Each one has actively participated in many scientific meetings on this subject and published papers in national and international journals. They run dedicated clinics on genital disorders, respectively, at the Departments of Dermatology of the Universities of Catania, Naples, and Milan.

The basic idea of this book is to describe vulvar disorders, rather than by standard classifications (infective, inflammatory, neoplastic, etc.), by the key elementary lesions (erythema, edema, vesicles, bullae, etc.) that characterize the clinical features. By doing so, the reader is provided with crucial clinical steps and emblematic and evocative pictures that may expedite the formulation of the correct diagnosis.

We hope that this publication may represent a useful and valuable tool for practicing physicians worldwide, who would benefit from reading it.

Basic Morphologic Terminology of Fundamental Lesions

Abrasion/Erosion: Lesion resulting from loss of the epithelium and superficial dermis, which usually heals with no scarring.

Abscess: Large, localized, superficial or, more often, deep-seated fluctuant accumulation of purulent material.

Bulla: Large, usually raised, tense or flaccid lesion filled with serous or hemorrhagic fluid resulting from intraepidermal or subepidermal cleavage.

Cyst: Cavity filled with fluid or semifluid material lined by a capsule.

Edema: Ill-defined skin swelling resulting from plasma exudation in the dermis; when only the papillary dermis is involved, it is called wheal.

Erythema: Blanchable reddening resulting from dilatation of dermal capillaries.

Keratosis: Epidermal thickening resulting in firmly adherent and nondetachable scales.

Lichenification: Epidermal thickening with prominent superficial markings resulting from repeated rubbing.

Nodule: Rounded, indurated and palpable lesion that may be either raised or embedded in the skin.

Papule: Circumscribed, raised and solid lesion of limited size.

Pigmentary change: Macule (if small) or patch (if large) characterized by a different color from its surrounding areas, with no other detectable surface alteration.

Plaque: Raised and solid palpable lesion with a relatively large surface area. Plaques may form by enlargement of a single papule or nodule or by confluence of multiple papules or nodules (papular/nodular plaques).

Pustule: Small circumscribed raised cavity containing purulent material.

Scaling: Superficial flakes that undergo desquamation as variably sized sheets of packed corneocytes.

Scarring: Fibrous tissue proliferation devoid of adnexal structures secondary to skin damage.

Ulcer: Lesion resulting from loss of the epithelium, superficial and deep dermis, which heals with scarring.

Vesicle: Small, usually raised lesion, primarily filled with clear fluid, resulting from intraepidermal or subepidermal cleavage.

1

Anatomy

Giuseppe Giuffrida and Giuseppe Micali

1.1 General Features

The vulva consists of the mons pubis, labia majora, labia minora, the hymen, the clitoris, the vestibule of the vagina, the urethral orifice, Skene's glands, Bartholin's glands, and the vestibular bulbs. The mons pubis, the perineum, and the labia share an ectodermal origin and have a keratinized, stratified, squamous epithelial structure with hair follicles, sebaceous glands, and sweat glands, similar to those of other skin sites. The degree of thickness of the vulvar skin epidermal keratinization progressively decreases from the outer part, the labia majora, to the inner part, the labia minora. The vulvar vestibule, conversely, is nonkeratinized and derived from the endodermal fold.

1.1.1 Mons Pubis

The mons pubis, or mons veneris, is the rounded eminence in front of the pubic symphysis that becomes covered by hair during puberty (A in Figure 1.1). It is characterized by a deep collection of adipose tissue.

1.1.2 Labia Majora

The labia majora are a pair of prominent longitudinal, cutaneous folds of fibro-adipose tissue that are homologous to the scrotum in males (B in Figure 1.1). They form the lateral boundaries of the vulva and are thicker anteriorly, where they join the mons pubis and form the anterior labial commissure (C in Figure 1.1). The posterior ends of the labia and the connecting skin between them form the posterior labial commissure. The labia majora are covered with a varying amount of hair and contain sebaceous, sweat eccrine, and apocrine glands.

1.1.3 Labia Minora

The labia minora are two thin pigmented folds of the vulva composed of a nonkeratinized stratified squamous epithelium (D in Figure 1.1). In a medial position to the labia majora, they are made up of loose connective tissue and blood vessels without any adipose tissue. Anteriorly, the labia minora are split into two parts: one part passes over the clitoris to form the prepuce, while the other joins with the contralateral one under the clitoris and forms the frenulum. Posteriorly, the labia minora blend with the medial surfaces of the labia majora. They are quite small in childhood, grow during puberty, and then become atrophic after menopause. The skin and mucosa are rich in sebaceous glands. Their inner aspect blends into the vulvar vestibule, and the junction of the squamous epithelium and the transitional epithelium forms Hart's line (black line in Figure 1.1).

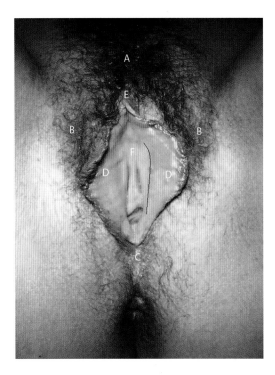

FIGURE 1.1   Anatomy of the vulva: (A) mons pubis; (B) labia majora; (C) anterior labial commissure; (D) labia minora; (E) clitoris; (F) vulvar vestibule; (black line) Hart's line corresponding to the boundary between the keratinized epithelium of the inner surface of the labia minora and the nonkeratinized transitional epithelium of the vulvar vestibule.

1.1.4 Clitoris

The clitoris is the erectile body of the vulva, similar to the corpora cavernosa of the penis. It is located beneath the anterior labial commissure, partially hidden between the anterior segments of the labia minora (E in Figure 1.1). It is composed of a body and a glans. The body consists of two corpora cavernosa covered by their ischiocavernous muscles. The glans is a small mass of erectile tissue that caps the body of the clitoris and is hidden by the prepuce.

1.1.5 Vulvar Vestibule

The vestibule is the cleft located posteriorly to the glans clitoridis and between the labia minora (F in Figure 1.1). It can be visualized by holding the labia minora apart. Hart's line marks the junction of the nonkeratinized epithelium of the vulvar vestibule and the keratinized epithelium of the inner surface of the labia minora (black line in Figure 1.1). Within the vestibule are the urethral meatus, the opening of Skene's paraurethral glands, the minor vestibular glands, the Bartholin's glands duct openings, and the lateral hymenal surface.

1.1.6 Urethral Meatus

The external urethral orifice is 4–6 mm in diameter and is immediately anterior to the vaginal orifice, approximately 2–3 cm beneath the glans clitoridis. The mucosa of the distal third of the urethra is lined by stratified squamous epithelium, whereas the proximal two-thirds are lined by stratified transitional epithelium.

1.1.7 Hymen

The hymen is a thin fold of mucous membrane situated at the entrance to the vagina. The shape of the prepubertal and/or virginal hymen varies, but it is most commonly annular or crescentic. It is very prominent in newborn children, due to maternal estrogens, and it regresses during childhood before the normal pubertal changes. Sexual intercourse and childbirth cause the disappearance of its larger part, leaving only remnants.

1.1.8 Vestibular Glands

The minor vestibular glands are situated around the hymenal ring. Among them, the largest ones are the Bartholin's glands, deeply located in the musculature.

1.1.9 Neurovascular Supply

The arterial blood supply comes from branches of the external and internal pudendal arteries. Lymph drains from the vulva into the medial group of superficial inguinal nodes on both the ipsilateral and contralateral sides. The sensory nerve system involves the genitofemoral nerve (L1 and L2) and the cutaneous branch of the ilioinguinal nerve (L1) for the anterior vulva, the pudendal nerve for the posterior part of the vulva, and the clitoris and the perineal branch of the posterior cutaneous nerve of the thigh for a small area of the posterior vulva.

Motor innervation of the perineal muscles is enabled by the pudendal nerve.

2

Erythema

Giuseppe Micali, Maria Rita Nasca, and Stefano Veraldi

2.1 Erythema

2.1.1 Intertrigo

Clinical aspect: Diffuse inguinal reddening and erythema (Figures 2.1.1 and 2.1.2) is a common finding, often more intense at the follicular openings with an overall uniformly "spotted" appearance; edema, oozing, malodorous maceration, and fissuring may ensue in acute stages, whereas lichenification and peripheral postinflammatory hyperpigmentation are typical of longstanding, chronic forms.

Definition: Nonspecific inflammatory eruption of inguinal folds.

Etiology: It can be precipitated by friction, occlusion, sweating, and obesity.

Epidemiology: It is common.

Clinical course: Soreness and itching are common symptoms. Recurrences after therapy are quite frequent in predisposed subjects.

Diagnosis: Clinical diagnosis is usually straightforward. Wood's light and skin swabs may be helpful for ruling out tinea cruris or erythrasma. A skin biopsy is seldom required in chronic forms to exclude other uncommon conditions, such as Hailey–Hailey disease.

Differential diagnosis: Candidiasis, bacterial infections, eczema (contact, atopic, and seborrheic dermatitis), Hailey–Hailey disease, inverse psoriasis, erythrasma, dermatophytosis, acrodermatitis entheropathica, Darier disease, and extramammary Paget disease.

Therapy: Treatment with a topical barrier and lenitive nongreasy creams and trauma avoidance is usually effective.

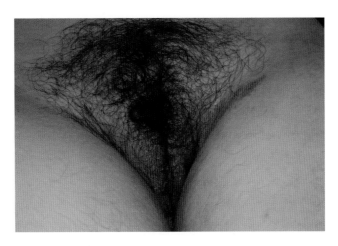

FIGURE 2.1.1   Acute intertrigo with prominent erythema of the inguinal folds.

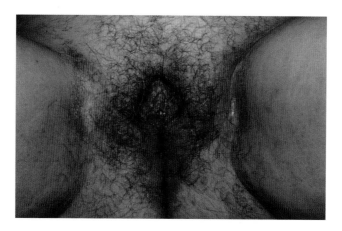

FIGURE 2.1.2   Acute intertrigo of inguinal folds extending to the perineal cleft.

Bibliography

Mistian P, Halm-Walters MV. Prevention and treatment of intertrigo in large skin folds of adults: A systematic review. *BMC Nurs* 2010;9:12.

Wolf R, Oumeish OY, Parish LC. Intertriginous eruption. *Clin Dermatol* 2011;29:173–9.

2.1.2 Inverse Psoriasis

Clinical aspect: On the vulva, inverse psoriasis more often appears as sharply demarcated, bright red, nonscaling and glazed patches that may be associated with pronounced vestibular erythema (psoriatic vestibulitis) (Figure 2.1.3). Inverse psoriasis may involve the genitocrural area with confluent, bright red, slightly scaling plaques on the labia majora and the mons pubis, and scattered, well-demarcated erythematous patches on the inner thigh (Figure 2.1.4). Smooth, well-defined erythematous patches involving the inguinal and gluteal folds in the napkin area (napkin psoriasis) as a result of the Koebner's phenomenon are also common findings in affected children (Figure 2.1.5). Symptoms are highly variable and may range from minimal discomfort to intense itching and/or burning. If pruritic, excoriations and lichenification due to scratching and rubbing may be observed.

Definition: Psoriasis is a chronic and/or relapsing erythemato-squamous inflammatory skin disorder. Inverse psoriasis is a clinical variant that is characterized by a predominant involvement of the great folds (including the genitocrural area).

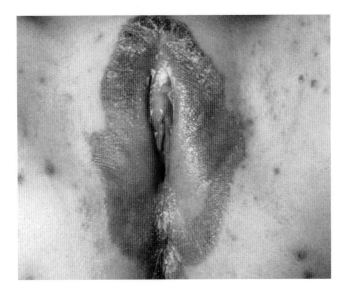

FIGURE 2.1.3 Typical sharply demarcated erythema in inverse psoriasis of the vulva.

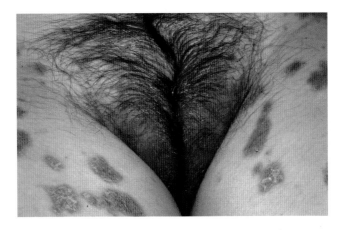

FIGURE 2.1.4 Vulvar psoriasis extending to the inguinal folds and inner thighs, where mild scaling may be apparent.

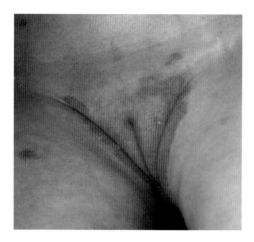

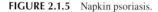

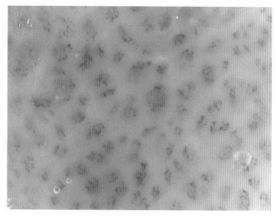

FIGURE 2.1.5   Napkin psoriasis.

FIGURE 2.1.6   Dermoscopy of inverse psoriasis: presence of dilated and tortuous capillaries with a "bushy" aspect.

Etiology: Its cause is unknown. Local factors (mechanical or chemical irritation from tight clothes, sexual intercourse, aggressive hygiene products, bacterial overgrowth, etc.) probably act as triggers capable of inducing the development of lesions in the genital area (Koebner's phenomenon).

Epidemiology: The genitocrural area is almost always affected in inverse psoriasis, although only a minority of patients show an exclusive genital involvement.

Clinical course: It runs a chronic and relapsing course, causing significant psychological effects. In case of bacterial or yeast superinfection, fissuration, oozing, and crusting may occur.

Diagnosis: It may be suggested by the presence of psoriatic lesions at other sites, typical nail findings or joint complaints, but traditionally requires histological confirmation. Recently, the use of videodermatoscopy, showing a dotted pattern at low magnifications ($\times 10 - \times 50$) and a typical "glomerular" or "bushy" capillary pattern at higher magnifications ($\times 100 - \times 400$), has been advocated as a useful noninvasive diagnostic tool (Figure 2.1.6).

Differential diagnosis: Candidiasis, bacterial infection, dermatophytosis, erythrasma, eczema (contact, atopic, and seborrheic dermatitis), Hailey–Hailey disease, lichen simplex chronicus, and Darier disease.

Therapy: In case of exclusive genital involvement, topical corticosteroids, in combination or not with vitamin D analogs (calcipotriol), or calcineurin inhibitors (pimecrolimus ointment or tacrolimus cream) may be useful. Systemic treatment is indicated when vulvar involvement occurs as part of a severe generalized psoriasis. Prevention of local traumas and accurate genital hygiene must be recommended in order to prevent bacterial and/or fungal secondary infections related to the disease itself or favored by the long-term use of topical steroids or immunomodulators.

Bibliography

Kapila S, Bradford J, Fischer G. Vulvar psoriasis in adults and children: A clinical audit of 194 cases and review of the literature. *J Low Genit Tract Dis* 2012;16:364–71.

Meeuwis KA, de Hullu JA, Massuger LF, van de Kerkhof PC, van Rossum MM. Genital psoriasis: A systematic literature review on this hidden skin disease. *Acta Derm Venereol* 2011;91:5–11.

Meeuwis KA, de Hullu JA, Van De Nieuwenhof HP, Evers AW, Massuger LF, van de Kerkhof PC, van Rossum MM. Quality of life and sexual health in patients with genital psoriasis. *Br J Dermatol* 2011;164:1247–55.

Meeuwis KA, van de Kerkhof PC, Massuger LF, de Hullu JA, van Rossum MM. Patients' experience of psoriasis in the genital area. *Dermatology* 2012;224:271–6.

Micali G, Lacarrubba F, Musumeci ML, Massimino D, Nasca MR. Cutaneous vascular patterns in psoriasis. *Int J Dermatol* 2010;49:249–56.

Musumeci ML, Lacarrubba F, Verzì AE, Micali G. Evaluation of the vascular pattern in psoriatic plaques in children using videodermatoscopy: an open comparative study. *Pediatr Dermatol* 2014;31:570-4.

2.1.3 Fixed Drug Eruption (Acute)

Clinical aspect: It frequently occurs in the genital area a few hours after drug intake as single or multiple sharply defined, round, or oval patches of erythema often showing a typical dusky red to violaceous hue (Figure 2.1.7); multiple lesions are more common in recurrences. Edema, blistering (Figure 2.1.8), and, eventually, oozing erosions may be observed during the acute stages (Figures 2.1.9 and 2.1.10). The main complaint is burning, but some patients are asymptomatic or have mild pruritus; eroded lesions are quite painful.

Definition: Genital fixed drug eruption is an adverse cell-mediated mucocutaneous reaction to an ingested drug that is characterized by a typical recurrence in the same site after retaking the offending drug.

Etiology: Any drug can cause fixed drug eruption by a direct cytotoxic immune-mediated effect. The most common causative agents include antibiotics (notably tetracycline), nonsteroidal anti-inflammatory agents, antiepileptics, and phenothiazines. Intake of the causative agent may occur via any route, including oral, rectal, or intravenous routes.

Epidemiology: It is frequent and may account for as much as 10%–20% of all drug eruptions. The actual frequency may be higher than current estimates, owing to the availability of a variety of over-the-counter medications and nutritional supplements that are known to elicit fixed drug eruptions. The most frequent localizations are the genitalia and the oral mucosa, but the genital skin is considered to be the most commonly involved site.

Clinical course: The eruption may occur as early as 30 minutes to 8 hours after ingestion of the drug in a previously sensitized individual, and persists if the offending drug is continued. After drug withdrawal, the lesions heal spontaneously in a few days or weeks leaving melanotic pigmentary changes as a residual dark brown to purplish postinflammatory hyperpigmentation. In case of reuptake of the same drug, the lesions relapse and worsen, leaving a postinflammatory pigmentation that increases at each repeated drug exposure.

Diagnosis: Diagnosis is usually made on clinical grounds, based on past medical history and clinical features. Blood studies are not considered useful, although eosinophilia is common with drug eruptions. Patch testing and oral provocation have been used to identify the suspected agent and check for cross-sensitivities to medications. Readministration of the drug may confirm the diagnosis, but should be avoided.

Differential diagnosis: Erythema multiforme, recurrent herpes simplex, intertrigo, bullous pemphigoid, and erosive lichen planus.

Therapy: After mandatory identification and discontinuation of the offending drug, treatment for fixed drug eruptions is otherwise symptomatic. Systemic antihistamines and topical corticosteroids may be effective for speeding up recovery. If secondary infection is suspected, antibiotics, antiseptics, and proper wound care are advised.

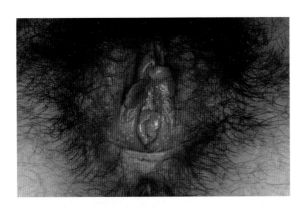

FIGURE 2.1.7 Acute fixed drug eruption.

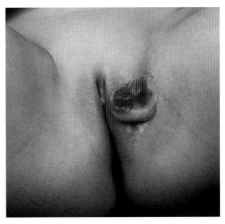

FIGURE 2.1.8 Secondary blistering in acute fixed drug eruption.

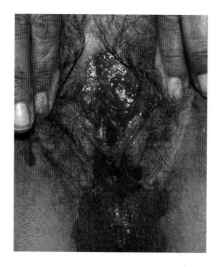

FIGURE 2.1.9   Secondary oozing, dark red erosions in acute fixed drug eruption.

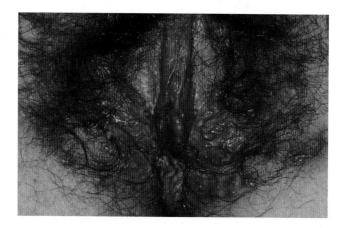

FIGURE 2.1.10   Blistering and oozing erosions with surrounding erythema in acute fixed eruption.

Bibliography

Fischer G. Vulvar fixed drug eruption. A report of 13 cases. *J Reprod Med* 2007;52:81–6.
Ozkaya-Bayazit E. Specific site involvement in fixed drug eruption. *J Am Acad Dermatol* 2003;49:1003–7.
Wain EM, Neill S. Fixed drug eruption of the vulva secondary to fluconazole. *Clin Exp Dermatol* 2008;33:
     784–5.

2.1.4 Trichomoniasis

Clinical aspect: The classical presentation is a profuse greenish-yellow, foul-smelling discharge exuding from the inflamed vaginal wall (Figure 2.1.11). The vagina may be tender and red, and the cervix usually shows a "strawberry" aspect, which is characterized by red dots due to tiny hemorrhagic lesions. Cervical involvement (Figure 2.1.12) is easily disclosed by iodine paint application (Figures 2.1.13 through 2.1.15). It can be associated with itching, soreness, and urinary disorders.

Definition: It is a common sexually transmitted vaginal infection.

Etiology: It is caused by a unicellular flagellate, *Trichomonas vaginalis.*

Epidemiology: It is more frequent in young women 20–29 years of age.

Clinical course: It is usually asymptomatic. If untreated, it can lead to pelvic inflammatory disease.

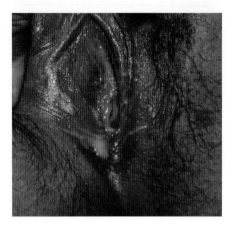

FIGURE 2.1.11   Evident vaginal discharge in trichomoniasis.

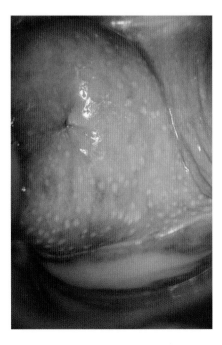

FIGURE 2.1.12   Cervical involvement in trichomoniasis.

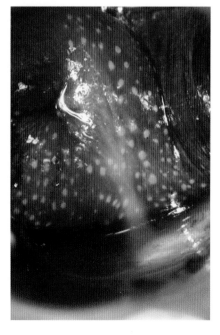

FIGURE 2.1.13   Cervical trichomoniasis after iodine paint application.

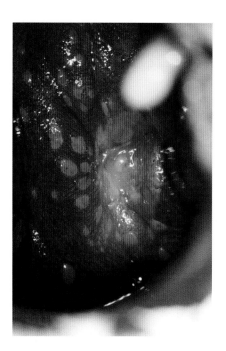

FIGURE 2.1.14   Cervical trichomoniasis after iodine paint application.

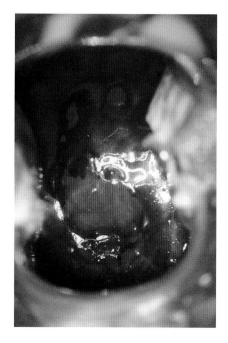

FIGURE 2.1.15   Cervical trichomoniasis after iodine paint application.

Diagnosis: The diagnosis has traditionally depended on microscopic observation and on culture. *Differential diagnosis*: Bacterial vaginosis, candidiasis, and chlamydial and gonococcal infections. *Therapy:* The main treatment is topical or oral metronidazole.

Bibliography

Azzam-W M, Cermeño-Vivas JR, Orellán-García Y, Penna SJ. Vulvovaginitis caused by *Candida* spp. and *Trichomonas vaginalis* in sexually active women. *Invest Clin* 2002;43:3–13.

Huppert JS. Trichomoniasis in teens: An update. *Curr Opin Obstet Gynecol* 2009;21:371–8.

Kassem HH, Majoud OA. Trichomoniasis among women with vaginal discharge in Benghazi city, Libya. *J Egypt Soc Parasitol* 2006;36:1007–16.

Mitchell L, Hussey J. *Trichomonas vaginalis*: An unusual presentation. *Int J STD AIDS* 2010;21:664–5.

2.1.5 Vulvar Vestibulitis

Clinical aspect: Tiny spots of vestibular erythema, ranging in diameter from 2 to 7 mm, surrounding the vulvovestibular gland openings and sometimes extending around the vulvar trigone may be observed (Figure 2.1.16). Typically, when a cotton-tipped applicator gently touches these areas, there is an exquisitely painful response. Rarely, small ulcerations may be detectable. Severe burning and pain on attempts at vaginal entry are consistently reported. There may be associated deep pain from secondary vaginismus, but examination of the vagina shows no vaginitis.

Definition: Complex pain syndrome, considered as a subset of vulvodynia, characterized by chronic increased sensitivity of the vestibular mucosa.

Etiology: Its cause is unknown. Possible factors that have been taken into consideration include contactans (irritants and chemicals), traumas and infections (subclinical human papillomavirus infection, chronic recurrent candidiasis, or chronic recurrent bacterial vaginosis), as well as genetic, hormonal, and psychological factors. Some investigators have postulated the existence of neurological (vestibular neural hyperplasia) or muscular causes (vaginal tightening due to hypertonic perivaginal muscles).

Epidemiology: The common age of occurrence is 35–40 years. Vulvar vestibulitis syndrome is considered the most common subtype of vulvodynia affecting premenopausal women.

Clinical course: Classically, there is marked tenderness, burning and pain when the involved area is touched, as with wiping, intercourse, or insertion of a tampon. The pain is enough to make intercourse uncomfortable or completely impossible, causing varying degrees of sexual dysfunction, followed by depression and anxiety.

Diagnosis: Diagnosis is clinical, after other causes of chronic vulvar pain have been ruled out. Point tenderness, not vulvovestibular erythema, is diagnostic, since the latter, without any genital discomfort, may be observed in normal women.

Differential diagnosis: Vulvovaginitis from different causes, vulvodynia, and vaginismus.

Therapy: Since vulvodynia is often a chronic condition, regular medical follow-up and referral to a support group are helpful for most patients. Suggested treatments include fluconazole, calcium citrate, tricyclic antidepressants, topical corticosteroids, physical therapy with biofeedback, surgery, or laser therapy.

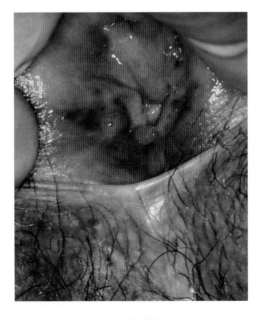

FIGURE 2.1.16 Spotted vestibular erythema in vulvar vestibulitis.

Bibliography

Bergeron S, Binik YM, Khalife S, Pagidas K. Vulvar vestibulitis syndrome: A critical review. *Clin J Pain* 1997;13:27–42.

Danby CS, Margesson LJ. Approach to the diagnosis and treatment of vulvar pain. *Dermatol Ther* 2010;23:485–504.

Edgardh K, Abdelnoor M. Vulvar vestibulitis and risk factors: A population-based case–control study in Oslo. *Acta Derm Venereol* 2007;87:350–4.

Tommola P, Unkila-Kallio L, Paavonen J. Surgical treatment of vulvar vestibulitis: A review. *Acta Obstet Gynecol Scand* 2010;89:1385–95.

2.2 Erythema plus Edema

2.2.1 Fungal/Bacterial Infection

Clinical aspect: Erythema and variable degrees of edema with purulent discharge are observed (Figures 2.2.1 through 2.2.3) and are usually associated with burning, pruritus, or both. Sometimes, marked skin scaling or follicular pustules may be present.

Definition: Bacterial/fungal vulvovaginitis is an acute inflammation due to trivial infectious agents.

Etiology: Common causative agents include both anaerobic and aerobic bacteria, such as *Staphylococcus* and *Streptococcus*. Mixed bacterial and yeast (*Candida*) infections are frequently observed. Commonly reported predisposing factors are irritation, occlusion, and maceration (intertrigo), with subsequent abnormal secondary bacterial colonization.

Epidemiology: It is considered frequent, although precise epidemiological data are currently unavailable.

Clinical course: The onset is usually abrupt. Symptoms may be so intense as to promptly induce the patient to seek medical advice. Erosions and crusting (Figure 2.2.4), ulcerations, and even abscess formation may sometimes ensue. Adenopathy and fever are frequently observed in such cases.

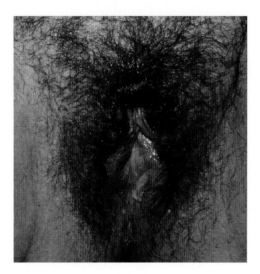

FIGURE 2.2.1 Vaginal discharge secondary to bacterial infection.

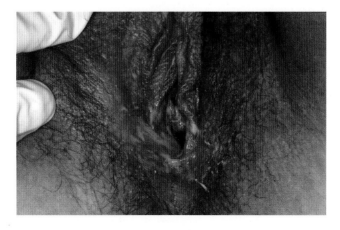

FIGURE 2.2.2 Mixed bacterial and yeast infection (candidiasis).

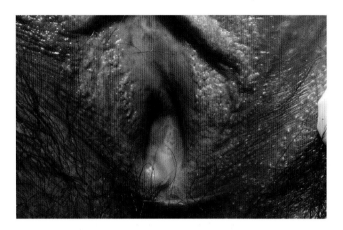

FIGURE 2.2.3   Mixed bacterial and candidal infection. Vulvar papillomatosis is also evident (see Section 7.1.2).

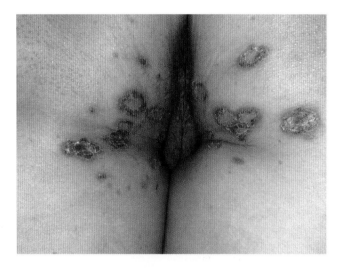

FIGURE 2.2.4   Erosions and crusting secondary to staphylococcal infection (impetigo) (Courtesy Professor Mario Pippione).

Diagnosis: A swab for bacterial culture is useful for identifying the involved bacteria and to specifically address the antibiotic therapy.

Differential diagnosis: Intertrigo, eczema (contact, atopic, and seborrheic dermatitis), Hailey–Hailey disease, inverse psoriasis, erythrasma, dermatophytosis, acrodermatitis entheropathica, and Darier disease.

Therapy: Topical and systemic antibiotics are indicated. Accurate genital hygiene with adequate antiseptic detergents should also be recommended.

Bibliography

Biggs WS, Williams RM. Common gynecologic infections. *Prim Care* 2009;36:33–51.

Eckert LO. Clinical practice. Acute vulvovaginitis. *N Engl J Med* 2006;355:1244–52.

Esim Buyukbayrak E, Kars B, Karsidag AY, Karadeniz BI, Kaymaz O, Gencer S, Pirimoglu ZM, Unal O, Turan MC. Diagnosis of vulvovaginitis: Comparison of clinical and microbiological diagnosis. *Arch Gynecol Obstet* 2010;282:515–9.

Sonnex C. Genital streptococcal infection in non-pregnant women: A case-note review. *Int J STD AIDS* 2013;24:447–8.

2.2.2 Candidiasis

Clinical aspect: Erythema and edema of the vestibule and of the labia minora and majora (Figures 2.2.5 and 2.2.6), typically spotted with whitish and loosely adherent thrush patches (Figure 2.2.7), are usually observed in the acute stages of the disease. Small peripheral erythematous papules, sometimes topped by whitish pustules and surrounded by erythema and a thick, white, curd-like vaginal discharge on the labial folds, vaginal opening, and cervix (Figure 2.2.8) may also be evident. Severe pruritus, soreness, irritation, burning on urination, and pain with intercourse are commonly reported symptoms.

Definition: It is a yeast mucosal infection that may also extend to vulvar skin and inguinal folds.

Etiology: Candida species are probably the most common causes of nonvenereal vulvovaginal infections. They are almost always present in the vaginal flora, but may in some instances overgrow and become pathogenic, causing an inflammatory disease. Although candidal infections may be sexually transmitted, the majority (85%–90%) of them are sporadic and caused by *Candida albicans*. The non-*albicans* species are frequently implicated in resistant cases.

Epidemiology: Although common in healthy subjects (it is reported in 40%–75% of sexually active women), vulvovaginal candidiasis may occur more frequently and severely in immune-compromised

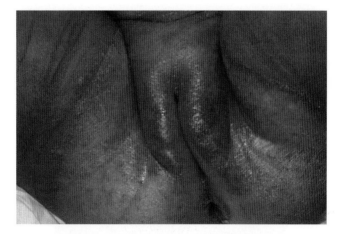

FIGURE 2.2.5　Candidiasis complicating napkin dermatitis.

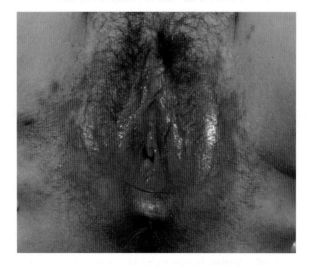

FIGURE 2.2.6　Acute candidiasis.

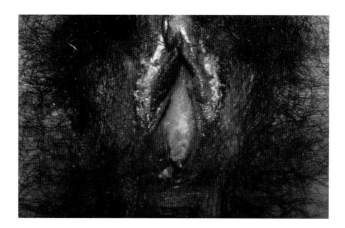

FIGURE 2.2.7   Loosely adherent thrush patches in acute candidiasis.

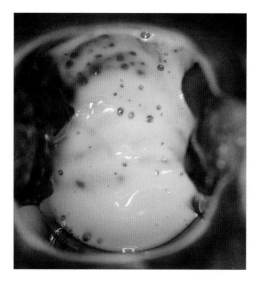

FIGURE 2.2.8   Cervical involvement with abundant white discharge in acute candidiasis.

women (HIV infection or during chronic treatment with topical/systemic corticosteroids or systemic chemotherapeutic agents and other immune-active drugs). Risk factors for candidiasis also include diabetes mellitus, the use of oral contraceptives and systemic antibiotics.

Clinical course: It usually runs an acute course, but relapses are common and sometimes lead to chronicization. In chronic vulvovaginal candidiasis, marked edema and lichenification of the vulva, sometimes with poorly defined margins and a grayish sheen made up of epithelial cells and organisms covering the area, are usually observed (Figure 2.2.9).

Diagnosis: It is often diagnosed by a focused physical examination of the external genitalia, vagina, and cervix, showing vulvovaginal inflammation with whitish plaques and a typical curd-like discharge. Bimanual examination should not elicit pain or tenderness and otherwise should be normal. Confirmation requires identification by direct microscopy of blastospores, hyphae, or pseudohyphae in saline and 10% potassium hydroxide preparations, or isolation of *Candida* sp. in microbiological cultures.

Differential diagnosis: Intertrigo, bacterial infections, eczema (contact, atopic, and seborrheic dermatitis), Hailey–Hailey disease, inverse psoriasis, erythrasma, dermatophytosis, acrodermatitis entheropatica, and Darier disease.

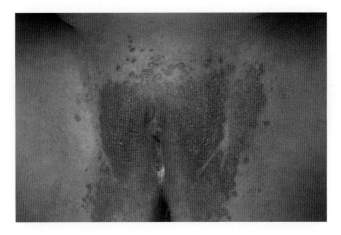

FIGURE 2.2.9   Erythema topped by white-grayish superficial scaling, marked lichenification and typical peripheral papules in chronic candidiasis complicating napkin dermatitis.

Therapy: Most strains of *C. albicans* causing uncomplicated sporadic vulvovaginal candidiasis exhibit sensitivity to azole-based topical antifungal agents. Effective treatment may also include oral agents, such as fluconazole or itraconazole. Whenever possible, treatment of sexual partners is recommended.

Bibliography

Chatwani AJ, Mehta R, Hassan S, Rahimi S, Jeronis S, Dandolu V. Rapid testing for vaginal yeast detection: A prospective study. *Am J Obstet Gynecol* 2007;196:309.

Donders G, Bellen G, Byttebier G, Verguts L, Hinoul P, Walckiers R, Stalpaert M, Vereecken A, Van Eldere J. Individualized decreasing-dose maintenance fluconazole regimen for recurrent vulvovaginal candidiasis (ReCiDiF trial). *Am J Obstet Gynecol* 2008;199:613.

Nyirjesy P. Vulvovaginal candidiasis and bacterial vaginosis. *Infect Dis Clin North Am* 2008;22:637–52.

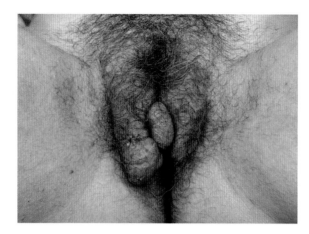

FIGURE 2.2.10　Erythema and prominent edema: erysipela.

2.2.3 Cellulitis/Erysipelas

Clinical aspect: The labia show signs of inflammation with erythema, edema, and painful red indurated plaques (Figure 2.2.10). The infection can be subtle when it involves only the vulva, with soreness, slight tenderness, and mild fever.

Definition: Cellulitis is an acute, spreading subcutaneous bacterial infection causing areas of hot, red, and tender skin.

Etiology: The most common causative agents are group A hemolytic streptococci and *Staphylococcus aureus*.

Epidemiology: It is rather uncommon and is more frequent in patients with diabetes and lymphedema.

Clinical course: In severe cases, the lesions may extend to the perineum, and eventually bullae and erosions may develop, with more severe local and/or systemic symptoms.

Diagnosis: The diagnosis is based on the clinical aspect.

Differential diagnosis: Contact dermatitis, urticaria/angioedema, herpes zoster, gangrene, and metastatic disease.

Therapy: Treatment with systemic antibiotics against *Streptococci* and *Staphylococci*.

Bibliography

Amankwah Y, Haefner H. Vulvar edema. *Dermatol Clin* 2010;28:765–77.

Aruch DB, Bhusal Y, Hamill RJ. Unusual cause of cellulitis in a patient with hepatitis C and cirrhosis. *Am J Med* 2011;124:e7–8.

Case records of the Massachusetts General Hospital. Weekly clinicopathology exercises. Case 26-1989. A 34-year-old woman with a history of Crohn's disease and recent vulvar cellulitis. *N Engl J Med* 1989;320:1741–7.

2.2.4 Gonorrhea

Clinical aspect: The usual appearance is of a mucopurulent endocervical and vaginal discharge. The vulva may be red, swollen and inflamed, but erythema and edema may be more evident at a chronic stage (Figures 2.2.11 through 2.2.14). Dysuria, burning, pruritus, and postcoital bleeding are common symptoms. Involvement of the Bartholin vestibular glands is frequent.

Definition: Gonorrhea is a sexually transmitted bacterial infection that usually affects the genitalia.

Etiology: It is caused by *Neisseria gonorrhoeae*, a Gram-negative intracellular diplococcus that may localize in the urethra and cervix in women and in the vaginal epithelium in prepubertal girls.

Epidemiology: It mainly affects young, sexually active adults.

Clinical course: It is almost asymptomatic in 80% of women.

Diagnosis: It is confirmed by the demonstration of *Neisseria gonorrhoeae* on Gram-stained smears and by its isolation through culture. Polymerase chain reaction (PCR) DNA probes may also be used.

Differential diagnosis: Trichomoniasis, bacterial vaginosis, candidiasis, and chlamydial infections.

Therapy: It is effectively treated with systemic antibiotics (penicillins, macrolides, and tetracyclines). The chance of antibiotic resistance and the consequent need for susceptibility testing to ensure radical treatment should be considered.

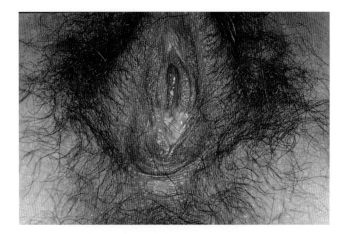

FIGURE 2.2.11   Erythema with mucopurulent vaginal discharge: gonorrhea.

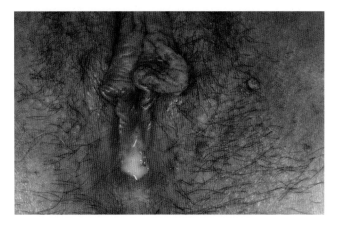

FIGURE 2.2.12   Gonorrhea; rounded papules recognizable as multiple condylomas are also evident (see Section 7.6.3).

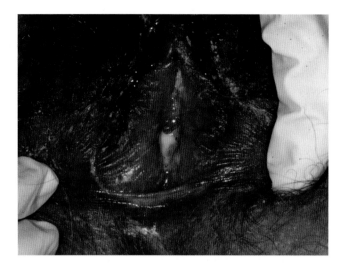

FIGURE 2.2.13   Intense erythema with mucopurulent vaginal discharge: gonorrhea.

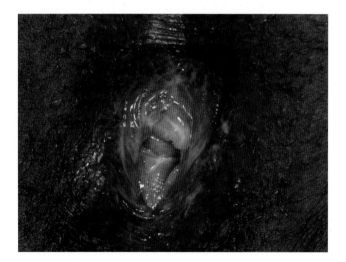

FIGURE 2.2.14   Gonorrhea in a dark-skinned patient.

Bibliography

Bignell C, Ison CA, Jungmann E. Gonorrhoea. *Sex Transm Infect* 2006;82 Suppl 4:iv6–9.
Woods CR. Gonococcal infections in neonates and young children. *Semin Pediatr Infect Dis* 2005;16:258–70.

2.2.5 Contact Dermatitis (Acute)

Clinical aspect: In acute contact dermatitis (CD), diffuse erythema and edema with ill-defined margins may involve the vulva and extend beyond the inguinal folds to the buttocks and thighs (possible association with regional intertrigo); folds may be spared in primary irritant CD (ICD), such as napkin dermatitis (Figures 2.2.15 and 2.2.16). Vulvar vestibulum involvement, with fissuring around the introitus, may sometimes be observed. Edema and scratch marks are frequent and may result in bacterial superinfection (Figures 2.2.17 and 2.2.18). Both burning and pruritus usually occur; however, the former is more often reported in primary ICD, whereas the latter is a common complaint in allergic CD (ACD). Dyspareunia is often reported in women with vestibular involvement.

Definition: It is a skin inflammation induced by an external agent acting as an irritant in ICD or an allergen in ACD. There is a spectrum from the acute stage, with mild local erythema or blistering and weeping lesions, to the chronic, late forms, with thick, fissured, and lichenified plaques.

Etiology: The inflammatory reaction is caused by physical or chemical agents acting by means of a direct nonimmunologic cytotoxic effect in the case of primary ICD or of a delayed, cell-mediated, type IV immune response in sensitized individuals in the case of ACD. Common products containing chemicals that may cause CD include soaps, menstrual pads, panty liners, toilet paper, diapers, fabric detergents, fabric softeners, feminine sprays, cosmetics, lubricants, spermicides, pessaries, and condoms; urine and feces are also frequent causes of vulvar ICD in infants and incontinent patients (napkin dermatitis), whereas saliva and semen can occasionally be allergenic. The topical medications that most often cause CD include benzocaine, hormonal creams, corticosteroids, topical antifungals, and antibiotics.

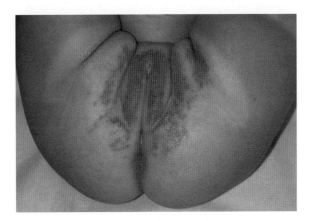

FIGURE 2.2.15 Erythema sparing skin folds in acute napkin dermatitis.

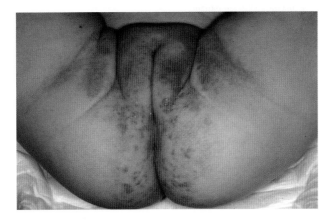

FIGURE 2.2.16 Erythema with ensuing scattered vesicles in acute napkin dermatitis.

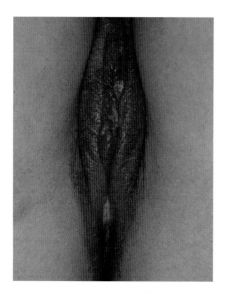

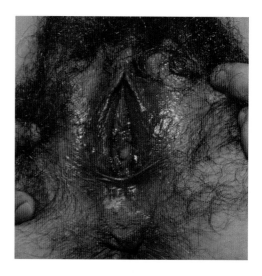

FIGURE 2.2.18   Acute contact dermatitis with bacterial superinfection.

FIGURE 2.2.17   Prominent edema due to acute contact dermatitis with bacterial superinfection.

Epidemiology: The incidence of vulvar CD in the general population is unknown; however, the reported incidence in a vulvar clinic was 20%–30% in the UK and 15% in Australia.

Clinical course: If the offending agent is identified and removed, ACD and ICD subside. If not, chronicization may ensue. Bacterial or yeast superinfections may complicate the clinical course.

Diagnosis: The diagnosis of vulvar CD is usually made by taking a detailed history and by careful physical examination. Patch tests may be helpful for identifying ACD; if they are negative and symptoms are reported to occur immediately after exposure, ICD should be considered. Biopsy may sometimes be required to rule out other conditions.

Differential diagnosis: Atopic dermatitis, seborrheic dermatitis, candidiasis, intertrigo, psoriasis, erythrasma, dermatophytosis, acrodermatitis entheropathica, Darier disease, and extramammary Paget disease.

Therapy: The cornerstone of the treatment of CD is the identification and removal of the causative irritant or allergen. Details of the patient's daily routine for genital hygiene should be reviewed. All patients should be instructed in proper vulvar care and advised to avoid all potential irritants, including friction from tight clothes and intercourse, use of spermicides, and artificial lubricants during the acute stage of the disease. Topical corticosteroids may be prescribed to decrease inflammation. Cold compresses and topical emollients may also be beneficial. Oral antihistamines may be used to help to alleviate pruritus. Superimposed bacterial and/or fungal infections should be ruled out and treated with antibiotics and antifungals. Barrier creams may be prescribed to minimize hazardous contact and prevent relapses.

Bibliography

Burrows LJ, Shaw HA, Goldstein AT. The vulvar dermatoses. *J Sex Med* 2008;5:276–83.

Crone AM, Stewart EJ, Wojnarowska F, Powell SM. Aetiological factors in vulvar dermatitis. *J Eur Acad Dermatol Venereol* 2000;14:181–6.

Haverhoek E, Reid C, Gordon L, Marshman G, Wood J, Selva-Nayagam P. Prospective study of patch testing in patients with vulval pruritus. *Australas J Dermatol* 2008;49:80–5.

Kint B, Degreef H, Dooms-Goossens A. Combined allergy to human seminal plasma and latex: Case report and review of the literature. *Contact Dermatitis* 1994;30:7–11.

Margesson LJ. Contact dermatitis of the vulva. *Dermatol Ther* 2004;17:20–7.

Nardelli A, Degreef H, Goossens A. Contact allergic reactions of the vulva: A 14-year review. *Dermatitis* 2004;15:131–6.

O'Gorman SM, Torgerson RR. Allergic contact dermatitis of the vulva. *Dermatitis* 2013;24:64–72.

Utaş S, Ferahbaş A, Yildiz S. Patients with vulval pruritus: Patch test results. *Contact Dermatitis* 2008;58:296–8.

2.3 Erythema plus Scales

2.3.1 Dermatophytosis

Clinical aspect: It appears as an often-pruritic erythematous skin eruption in the hair-bearing portion of the vulva (Figures 2.3.1 and 2.3.2), with characteristic annular scaling borders that slowly grow centrifugally over a number of weeks (Figures 2.3.3 and 2.3.4). It may extend bilaterally and symmetrically to the inguinal creases (Figure 2.3.5), and around the buttock area. Erythematous papules, maceration, and pustules (Figure 2.3.6) may sometimes be observed.

Definition: It is a superficial fungal infection, also known as tinea cruris and ringworm, which usually involves the groin and may extend to the genitalia.

Etiology: Causative agents include *Epidermophyton floccosum*, *Trichophyton rubrum*, and *Trichophyton mentagrophytes*.

Epidemiology: It mostly affects young adults. Women are less commonly affected than men. A primary pubic and/or vulvar localization of dermatophytosis has rarely been reported, as it is usually linked to spread from inguinal folds. It can be transmitted from a sexual partner or via autoinoculation (the patient may have tinea pedis and/or onychomycosis at the same time as a source of infection). It is worse in those wearing tight synthetic clothing.

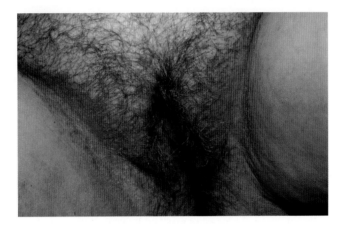

FIGURE 2.3.1 Inguinal creases showing erythema with marginal scaling: dermatophytosis.

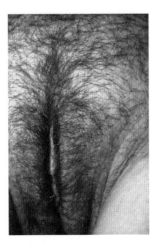

FIGURE 2.3.2 Roundish erythematous and scaling eruption (ringworm): dermatophytosis.

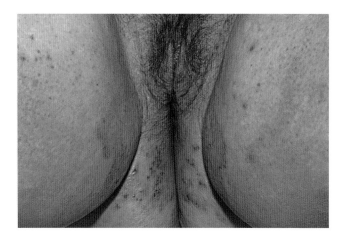

FIGURE 2.3.3   Prominent annular borders: dermatophytosis.

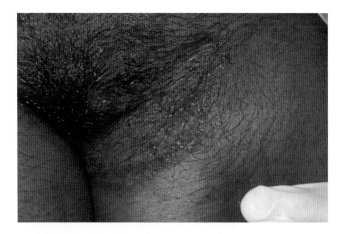

FIGURE 2.3.4   Dermatophytosis in a dark-skinned patient.

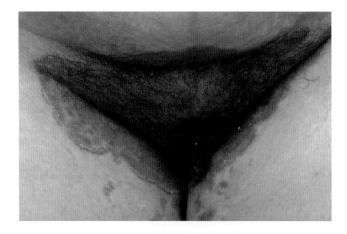

FIGURE 2.3.5   Progressively enlarging patch of erythema with sharply marginated and scaling borders: dermatophytosis (Courtesy Professor Mario Pippione).

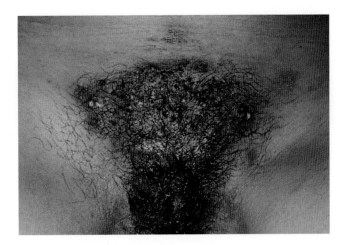

FIGURE 2.3.6 Scattered pustules from follicular involvement in a case of dermatophytosis with marked inflammation.

Clinical course: It is usually eradicated with adequate treatment, although recurrences may occur. Inappropriate treatment with topical corticosteroids may cause the development of tinea incognita, which is a misdiagnosed atypical fungal infection.

Diagnosis: The clinical pattern alone can be diagnostic, but is better confirmed by microscopic diagnosis with 10% potassium hydroxide and/or culture from a peripheral scale.

Differential diagnosis: Candidiasis, bacterial infections, eczema (contact, atopic, and seborrheic dermatitis), Hailey–Hailey disease, inverse psoriasis, erythrasma, intertrigo. acrodermatitis entheropathica, Darier disease, and extramammary Paget disease.

Therapy: Topical medications, which are effective for erythema and scaling without pustules or papules, include antifungal creams containing azoles or allylamines. Extensive forms, thick plaques, or evidence of follicular involvement may require oral antimycotic therapy.

Bibliography

Barile F, Filotico R, Cassano N. Pubic and vulvar inflammatory tinea due to *Trichophyton mentagrophytes*. *Int J Dermatol* 2006;45:1369–70.

Chang SE, Lee DK, Choi JH, Moon KC, Koh JK. Majocchi's granuloma of the vulva caused by *Trichophyton mentagrophytes*. *Mycoses* 2005;48:382–4.

Margolis DJ, Weinberg JM, Tangoren IA, Cheney RT, Johnson BL Jr. Trichophytic granuloma of the vulva. *Dermatology* 1998;197:69–70.

Pinto V, Marinaccio M, Serratì A, D'Addario V, Saracino V, De Marzo P. Kerion of the vulva. Report of a case and review of the literature. *Minerva Ginecol* 1993;45:501–5.

2.3.2 Contact Dermatitis (Chronic)

Clinical aspect: Desquamation (scaling), dryness (xerosis), and lichenification superimposed on an ill-defined patch of erythema clinically characterize chronic CD (Figures 2.3.7 and 2.3.8). Excoriations, fissures, and sometimes ulcerations may be observed within the thick and lichenified plaques. Intense itching is frequently reported.

Definition: It is a chronic inflammatory skin reaction related to persistent primary ICD or ACD.

Etiology: The inflammatory reaction is caused by physical or chemical agents acting by means of a direct nonimmunologic cytotoxic effect in the case of primary ICD or of a delayed, cell-mediated, type IV immune response in sensitized individuals in the case of ACD.

Epidemiology: The reported incidence of either acute or chronic CD ranges from 15% (Australia) to 30% (UK) in vulvar clinics.

Clinical course: Bacterial or yeast superinfections may occur. Severe and persistent itching may be very stressful for patients, causing sleep disturbances and significant psychological discomfort.

Diagnosis: The diagnosis of vulvar CD is usually made by taking a detailed history and by careful physical examination. Patch tests may be helpful for identifying ACD; if they are negative and symptoms

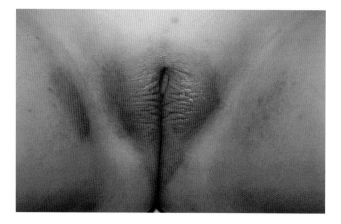

FIGURE 2.3.7 Prominent lichenification sparing the inguinal folds in chronic contact (napkin) dermatitis.

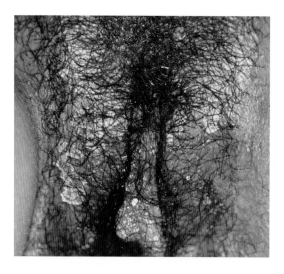

FIGURE 2.3.8 Abudant whitish scaling in chronic contact dermatitis.

are reported to occur immediately after exposure, ICD should be considered. Biopsy may sometimes be required to rule out other conditions.

Differential diagnosis: Atopic dermatitis, candidiasis, psoriasis, lichen sclerosus, lichen simplex chronicus, erythrasma, dermatophytosis, acrodermatitis entheropathica, Darier disease, and extramammary Paget disease.

Therapy: The cornerstone of the treatment of CD is the identification and removal of the causative irritant or allergen. Details of the patient's daily routine for genital hygiene should be reviewed. All patients should be instructed in proper vulvar care and advised to avoid all potential irritants and allergens (harsh soaps, fabric detergents and softeners, flavored cosmetics, sprays, menstrual pads or toilet paper, lubricants, spermicides, and unnecessary topical drugs). Topical emollients and corticosteroids may be prescribed to decrease inflammation. Regular use of barrier creams should also be suggested. Superimposed bacterial and/or fungal infections should be ruled out and treated with antibiotics and antifungals. Oral antihistamines or low-dose tricyclic antidepressants may be used to help to alleviate pruritus and facilitate sleep. Short courses of oral corticosteroids, cyclosporine, and topical calcineurin inhibitors may represent alternative options in severe and/or resistant cases of ACD.

Bibliography

Burrows LJ, Shaw HA, Goldstein AT. The vulvar dermatoses. *J Sex Med* 2008;5:276–83.

Crone AM, Stewart EJ, Wojnarowska F, Powell SM. Aetiological factors in vulvar dermatitis. *J Eur Acad Dermatol Venereol* 2000;14:181–6.

Haverhoek E, Reid C, Gordon L, Marshman G, Wood J, Selva-Nayagam P. Prospective study of patch testing in patients with vulval pruritus. *Australas J Dermatol* 2008;49:80–5.

Margesson LJ. Contact dermatitis of the vulva. *Dermatol Ther* 2004;17:20–7.

Nardelli A, Degreef H, Goossens A. Contact allergic reactions of the vulva: A 14-year review. *Dermatitis* 2004;15:131–6.

O'Gorman SM, Torgerson RR. Allergic contact dermatitis of the vulva. *Dermatitis* 2013;24:64–72.

Utaş S, Ferahbaş A, Yildiz S. Patients with vulval pruritus: Patch test results. *Contact Dermatitis* 2008;58:296–8.

2.3.3 Atopic Dermatitis

Clinical aspect: The genital area may become extremely itchy and inflamed (Figure 2.3.9). Mild erythema, xerosis, and fine scaling with ill-defined margins symmetrically affect the labia majora and—less frequently—the labia minora and inner thighs. Minute and fragile scattered vesicles that easily erode frequently ensue (Figure 2.3.10). Consequent weeping and—occasionally—superimposed bacterial infections result in honey-colored crusting. In chronic forms, repeated scratching may lead to lichenification and hyperpigmentation. Itching and burning are common symptoms.

Definition: Chronically relapsing inflammatory dermatosis, predominantly occurring in patients with a personal or family history of atopy, characterized by pruritus, eczema, xerosis (dry skin), and lichenification.

Etiology: It is unknown, but related to cutaneous hypersensitivity, IgE overproduction, and defective cell-mediated immunity. Genetic factors are likely, since it is often seen in multiple members of the same family. Several environmental conditions may trigger or worsen the disease, including cold weather, exposure to aggressive detergents, tight clothing, and seasonal allergies.

Epidemiology: It is very common, accounting for approximately 20% of all dermatologic referrals in some series; in addition, its incidence and prevalence appear to be increasing. Genital localization is considered rare.

Clinical course: It is a chronic disease that most often starts in early infancy but may sometimes persist or relapse into adulthood.

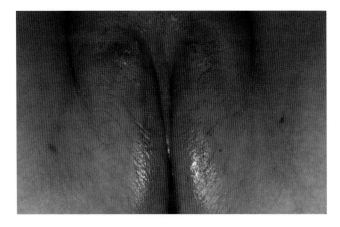

FIGURE 2.3.9   Vulvar pruritic inflammation: atopic dermatitis.

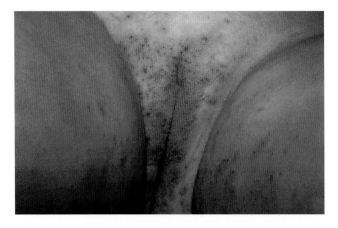

FIGURE 2.3.10   Erythema with superimposed blistering and crusting in atopic dermatitis.

Diagnosis: Currently, there is no single specific diagnostic test available, although dermoscopy may be useful to rule out psoriasis. Past medical history and clinical aspect generally prompt the correct diagnosis.

Differential diagnosis: Inverse psoriasis, seborrheic dermatitis, contact dermatitis, candidiasis, bacterial infections, erythrasma, dermatophytosis, lichen simplex chronicus, and acrodermatitis entheropathica.

Therapy: The primary treatment involves prevention by avoiding or minimizing exposure to environmental triggers. Effective topical treatments include emollients, corticosteroids, and topical calcineurin inhibitors (pimecrolimus cream and tacrolimus ointment). Topical or systemic antibiotics should be used in case of bacterial superinfection. Oral antihistamines may be helpful for controlling night-time scratching.

Bibliography

Beltrani VS. Atopic dermatitis in adults. *Dermatitis* 2012;23:52–3.

Cookson H, Smith C. Systemic treatment of adult atopic dermatitis. *Clin Med* 2012;12:172–6.

Crone AM, Stewart EJ, Wojnarowska F, Powell SM. Aetiological factors in vulvar dermatitis. *J Eur Acad Dermatol Venereol* 2000;14:181–6.

Denby KS, Beck LA. Update on systemic therapies for atopic dermatitis. *Curr Opin Allergy Clin Immunol* 2012;12:421–6.

Fischer G. Chronic vulvitis in pre-pubertal girls. *Australas J Dermatol* 2010;51:118–23.

García-Avilés C, Carvalho N, Fernández-Benítez M. Allergic vulvovaginitis in infancy: Study of a case. *Allergol Immunopathol* 2001;29:137–40.

2.3.4 Seborrheic Dermatitis

Clinical aspect: Genital lesions are usually observed in the setting of a more generalized disease. Dry to greasy scales superimposed on well-defined roundish, multiple, confluent, erythematous, and yellowish plaques mainly affect the labia majora and mons pubis (Figures 2.3.11 and 2.3.12) and sometimes extend to the gluteal cleft and thighs. Mild pruritus is common, but some patients are asymptomatic.

Definition: It is a chronic relapsing inflammatory dermatosis with a predilection for areas that are rich in sebaceous glands.

Etiology: Although the exact cause is still unclear, it is evidently related to sebaceous gland activity, yeast hyperproliferation (*Pityrosporum*), and immune function. It may be worsened by seasonal climatic changes, psychological or physical stress (systemic illness and debilitation), immunosuppression (especially HIV), or neurological disorders (Parkinson's disease or stroke).

Epidemiology: It is common, with a prevalence of approximately 1%–2% in the general population, and can affect patients from infancy to old age. Genital localization is uncommon and more often observed in women than men.

Clinical course: In infants, it usually disappears spontaneously, but may persist and become generalized in immunodeficient subjects. In adolescents and adults, it has a chronic and relapsing course, and there is usually no strategy that stops it permanently.

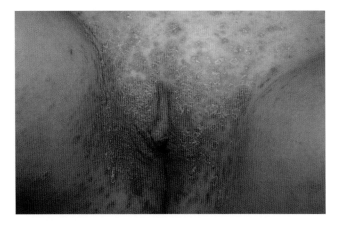

FIGURE 2.3.11   Dry to greasy scales with underlying rounded and confluent patches of erythema in seborrheic dermatitis.

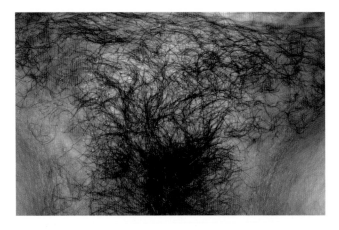

FIGURE 2.3.12   Erythema and scaling on the mons pubis due to seborrheic dermatitis.

Diagnosis: The diagnosis can be made based on the medical history and physical examination. Inspection of other seborrheic areas is usually helpful for suggesting the correct diagnosis. Direct microscopical examination of a specimen of a superficial skin scraping prepared with potassium hydroxide may be useful for ruling out other fungal infections. When the diagnosis is unclear, a skin biopsy is suggested, although the histological findings are not specific.

Differential diagnosis: Conditions commonly confused with seborrheic dermatitis include psoriasis, bacterial/fungal infections (including candidiasis, erythrasma, and dermatophytosis), and atopic and contact dermatitis.

Therapy: Both antifungal and anti-inflammatory preparations (creams, foams, or lotions) have been used to treat seborrheic dermatitis effectively and safely. Intermittent applications of low-potency topical steroids may also be useful.

Bibliography

Crone AM, Stewart EJ, Wojnarowska F, Powell SM. Aetiological factors in vulvar dermatitis. *J Eur Acad Dermatol Venereol* 2000;14:181–6.

Dessinioti C, Katsambas A. Seborrheic dermatitis: Etiology, risk factors, and treatments: Facts and controversies. *Clin Dermatol* 2013;31:343–51.

Gaitanis G, Magiatis P, Hantschke M, Bassukas ID, Velegraki A. The *Malassezia* genus in skin and systemic diseases. *Clin Microbiol Rev* 2012;25:106–41.

Sampaio AL, Mameri AC, Vargas TJ, Ramos-e-Silva M, Nunes AP, Carneiro SC. Seborrheic dermatitis. *An Bras Dermatol* 2011;86:1061–71.

Schmidt JA. Seborrheic dermatitis: A clinical practice snapshot. *Nurse Pract* 2011;36:32–7.

Schwartz RA, Janusz CA, Janniger CK. Seborrheic dermatitis: An overview. *Am Fam Physician* 2006;74: 125–130.

3

Edema

Stefano Veraldi, Maria Rita Nasca, and Giuseppe Micali

3.1 Edema

3.1.1 Angioedema

Clinical aspect: It presents with a sudden onset of circumscribed and evanescent areas of edema involving both the skin and the mucosa of the genital area (Figures 3.1.1 and 3.1.2). It may be isolated or occur as a manifestation of a generalized urticaria. It may sometimes be painful.

Clinical course: It is characterized by recurrent episodes.

Definition: It is an acute, inflammatory disorder characterized by the rapid onset of edema involving cutaneous, subcutaneous, and mucosal tissues.

Etiology: It can be caused by a localized allergic reaction, more often in subjects with a latex allergy (condoms or diaphragms) or who are sensitized to their partner's genital discharge. An inherited autosomal dominant variant resulting from a deficiency or a dysfunction of the C1 inhibitor is also well known.

Epidemiology: Genital angioedema is rare.

Diagnosis: The diagnosis of angioedema is clinical. Laboratory investigations for C4, C1q, and C1 inhibitor (antigenic and functional) blood levels should be performed to rule out hereditary angioedema. Testing for allergy is also recommended.

Differential diagnosis: Urticaria, cellulitis/erysipelas, contact dermatitis, herpes zoster, and gangrene.

Therapy: The treatment of idiopathic angioedema is the same as that of urticaria and includes the use of systemic antihistamines and corticosteroids. Hereditary angioedema requires proper prophylactic strategies and pharmacological management of the acute attacks.

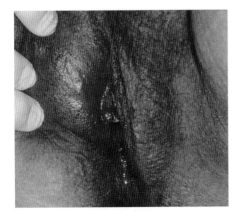

FIGURE 3.1.1 Angioedema.

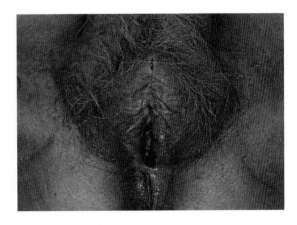

FIGURE 3.1.2 Angioedema.

Bibliography

Beckmann M, Mühlenstedt D, Happle R. Pregnancy and delivery combined with hereditary angioneurotic edema (author's transl). *Geburtshilfe Frauenheilkd* 1979;39:338–40.

Caballero T, Farkas H, Bouillet L, Bowen T, Gompel A, Fagerberg C, Bjökander J et al., C-1-INH Deficiency Working Group. International consensus and practical guidelines on the gynecologic and obstetric management of female patients with hereditary angioedema caused by C1 inhibitor deficiency. *J Allergy Clin Immunol* 2012;129:308–20.

Dhairyawan R, Harrison R, Buckland M, Hourihan M. Hereditary angioedema: An unusual cause of genital swelling presenting to a genitourinary medicine clinic. *Int J STD AIDS* 2011;22:356–7.

Hardy F, Ngwingtin L, Bazin C, Babinet P. Hereditary angioneurotic edema and pregnancy. *J Gynecol Obstet Biol Reprod* 1990;19:65–8.

3.1.2 Lymphedema

Clinical aspect: The first symptom of lymphedema is either unilateral (Figure 3.1.3) or bilateral (Figure 3.1.4) nontender, pitting edema.

Definition: It is an abnormal collection of protein-rich fluid in the interstitium resulting from an obstruction of lymphatic drainage with consequent swelling of the soft tissues.

Etiology: It can be primary or secondary. In primary lymphedema, patients have a congenital defect in the lymphatic system; this is more often associated with other anomalies and/or genetic disorders (yellow nail syndrome, Turner syndrome, and xanthomatosis). Secondary lymphedema may be due to a neoplasm obstructing the lymphatic system, recurrent episodes of lymphangitis and/or cellulitis, obesity, trauma or surgery, and/or radiation therapy. Filariasis is another common cause of massive genital lymphedema in underdeveloped tropical countries.

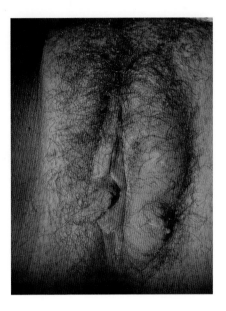

FIGURE 3.1.3 Unilateral lymphedema.

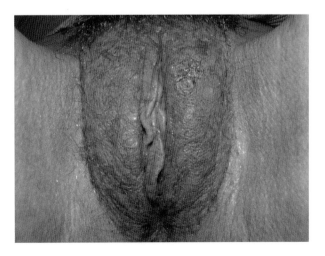

FIGURE 3.1.4 Bilateral lymphedema.

Epidemiology: Primary forms are uncommon, whereas acquired forms tend to be more frequent.

Clinical course: With time, subcutaneous tissue sclerosis may ensue. These patients are at higher risk of bacterial superinfections.

Diagnosis: The diagnosis is clinical; however, laboratory investigations may sometimes be helpful to rule out some causes of secondary lymphedema.

Differential diagnosis: Urticaria/angioedema, cellulitis/erysipelas, contact dermatitis, herpes zoster, gangrene, and metastatic disease.

Therapy: The aim is to restore function, reduce physical and psychological discomfort, and prevent the development of superinfections.

Bibliography

Adesiyun AG, Samaila MO. Huge filarial elephantiasis vulvae in a Nigerian woman with subfertility. *Arch Gynecol Obstet* 2008;278:597–600.

Baeyens L, Vermeersch E, Bourgeois P. Bicyclist's vulva: Observational study. *BMJ* 2002;325:138–9.

Bourgeault E, Giroux L. An approach to the treatment of vulvar lymphedema. *J Cutan Med Surg* 2011;15:61–2.

Eva LJ, Narain S, Luesley DM. Idiopathic vulval lymphoedema. *J Obstet Gynaecol* 2007;27:748–9.

Fadare O, Brannan SM, Arin-Silasi D, Parkash V. Localized lymphedema of the vulva: A clinicopathologic study of 2 cases and a review of the literature. *Int J Gynecol Pathol* 2011;30:306–13.

Orosz Z, Lehoczky O, Szoke J, Pulay T. Recurrent giant fibroepithelial stromal polyp of the vulva associated with congenital lymphedema. *Gynecol Oncol* 2005;98:168–71.

Plaza JA, Requena L, Kazakov DV, Vega E, Kacerovska D, Reyes G, Michal M, Suster S, Sangueza M. Verrucous localized lymphedema of genital areas: Clinicopathologic report of 18 cases of this rare entity. *J Am Acad Dermatol* 2014;71:320–6.

Talwar A, Puri N, Sandhu HP. Vulval lymphoedema following pulmonary tuberculosis. *Int J STD AIDS* 2009;20:437–9.

3.2 Edema plus Ulcers

3.2.1 Lymphogranuloma Venereum

Clinical aspect: Following sexual contact with an infected subject, after an incubation period of 3–30 days, small, inconspicuous, painless, and short-lived erosions or shallow ulcers, sometimes preceded by little blisters or papules, appear in the genital area corresponding to the portal of entry of the infection. These primary lesions tend to heal spontaneously within 1 week and often go unnoticed. Subsequently, acute unilateral or bilateral inguinal lymphadenitis ensues. Multiple inguinal nodes are usually affected. Massive inguinal swelling often shows a characteristic groove (Greenblatte sign) due to the Poupart's ligament between inguinal and femoral enlarged lymph nodes. Chronic inflammation leads to the formation of ulcerations and fistulae, with drainage of purulent material through the skin (buboes), and to destruction of the local lymphatic drainage system, resulting in genital lymphatic edema (elephantiasis) (Figure 3.2.1). General symptoms, such as fever, malaise, headache, arthralgias, diarrhea, and lower abdominal pain, are often present.

Definition: It is a chronic, long-term bacterial infection of the lymphatic system affecting the genital area. It is also known as Durand–Nicolas–Favre disease.

Etiology: It is a sexually transmitted disease that may be caused by three different serotypes (L1, L2, and L3) of *Chlamydia trachomatis.*

Epidemiology: It is endemic in tropical and subtropical areas of Africa, South-East Asia, Latin America, and the Caribbean. Until 2003, sporadic cases were reported in Europe and North America.

Clinical course: Untreated, lymphogranuloma venereum persists for several months or years. Possible complications, besides genital elephantiasis, include anal stenosis and rectal strictures due to the involvement of perirectal lymph nodes.

Diagnosis: It is achieved by exclusion of other causes of lymphadenopathy and is confirmed by blood complement fixation testing and by laboratory investigations aimed at *C. trachomatis* detection (culture, microimmunofluorescence, and PCR).

Differential diagnosis: Chancroid, granuloma inguinale, herpes simplex, syphilis, Crohn's disease (CD), and hidradenitis suppurativa.

Therapy: Oral antibiotics are commonly prescribed to treat this disease. The treatment of choice is doxycycline, although tetracycline, erythromycin, and azithromycin are also effective. Incision and surgical drainage of purulent discharge above the inguinal ligament may minimize symptoms.

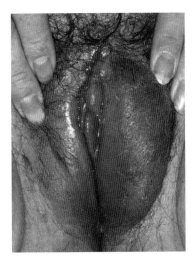

FIGURE 3.2.1   Massive labial lymphedema with ulceration: lymphogranuloma venereum.

Bibliography

Amankwah Y, Haefner H. Vulvar edema. *Dermatol Clin* 2010;28:765–77.

Bébéar C, de Barbeyrac B. Genital *Chlamydia trachomatis* infections. *Clin Microbiol Infect* 2009;15:4–10.

Gupta S, Ajith C, Kanwar AJ, Sehgal VN, Kumar B, Mete U. Genital elephantiasis and sexually transmitted infections—Revisited. *Int J STD AIDS* 2006;17:157–65.

Kapoor S. Re-emergence of lymphogranuloma venereum. *J Eur Acad Dermatol Venereol* 2008;22:409–16.

Manavi K. A review on infection with *Chlamydia trachomatis*. *Best Pract Res Clin Obstet Gynaecol* 2006;20:941–51.

3.2.2 Crohn's Disease

Clinical aspect: Genital Crohn's disease (CD) can present in several different forms, extending to the inguinal, perineal, and perianal regions and involving the vulva in women. Anogenital patterns of CD include the following: contiguous (in which skin lesions follow direct extensions from areas near the affected bowel), metastatic (in which skin sites distant from the gastrointestinal tract are involved), and nonspecific mucocutaneous lesions. Genital lesions often appear as nonhealing ulcers, but they can present as a papule, a plaque, or swelling. In vulvar CD, partial or massive labial edema, eventually leading to labial hypertrophy, which may or may not be inflammatory, is frequently observed (Figure 3.2.2). Although superimposed coalescing pustules may occasionally occur, single or multiple erosions or ulcers of variable extension and depth usually represent the most common associated findings (Figures 3.2.3 and 3.2.4). Distinctive ulcerations associated with this condition are the so-called "knife cut" linear fissures, which are located along the labiocrural fold. Deep single necrotic ulcers, eventually progressing to perianal or rectovaginal fistulae, may also develop. In some patients, raised growths mimicking anogenital warts (pyostomatitis vegetans) may be observed (Figure 3.2.5). Skin ulcers may be very painful, causing considerable

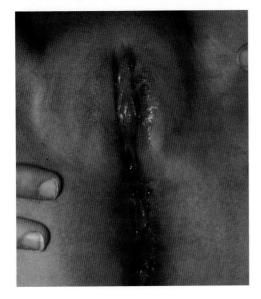

FIGURE 3.2.2 Labial edema: Crohn's disease.

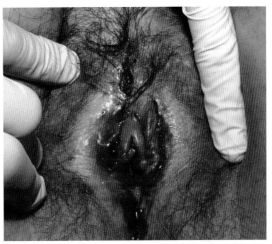

FIGURE 3.2.3 Multiple erosions with vulvar edema: Crohn's disease.

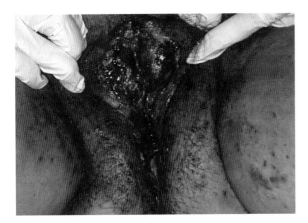

FIGURE 3.2.4 Ulcerative lesions with vulvar edema: Crohn's disease.

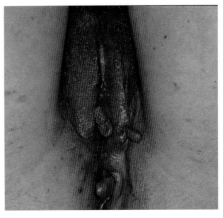

FIGURE 3.2.5 Raised vegetations with prominent infiltrated edema: Crohn's disease.

discomfort and impairing the quality of life. Interestingly, the severity of the cutaneous findings may not correlate with the severity of the bowel symptoms (abdominal pain, chronic diarrhea, vomiting, and wasting or weight loss).

Definition: It is a chronic, granulomatous, inflammatory bowel disease that can occasionally involve the vulva and groin, either primarily or secondarily.

Etiology: It is unknown. Proposed causes include a disturbed immunologic reaction to an unrecognized intestinal infectious agent in a genetically predisposed individual. Psychological factors are reported to represent potential triggers for the periodic exacerbations of the disease.

Epidemiology: CD commonly occurs between the ages of 20–30 years. Of women with this disorder, 2% have associated vulvar involvement, usually presenting after the onset of bowel symptoms, although genital involvement has been reported to precede bowel symptoms by 3 months to 8 years in 20% of patients.

Clinical course: This is a long-term disorder, with little or no evidence of spontaneous remission. Healing of anogenital lesions usually occurs with scarring.

Diagnosis: Diagnosis may be challenging, especially when systemic symptoms develop after the onset of the skin lesions. It is based on clinical history and histological findings, showing in the dermis typical noncaseating granulomas arranged in a perivascular distribution.

Differential diagnosis: Hidradenitis suppurativa, aphthosis, and Behçet disease, lymphogranuloma venereum, chancroid, granuloma inguinale, herpes simplex, syphilis, sarcoidosis, and tuberculosis.

Therapy: Therapy depends on the extent of the involvement of the perineal area and the associated bowel disease. Prospective studies or case series with long follow-up data are still missing for guiding the treatment of this condition. Treatment options include prolonged oral courses of metronidazole and systemic immunosuppressive therapy, such as corticosteroids or azathioprine. Sulfasalazine, tetracyclines, dapsone, and hyperbaric oxygen may also be useful, and there are promising published data on the efficacy of infliximab. Surgery remains restricted to medical treatment failures or the resection of unsightly lesions.

Bibliography

Barret M, de Parades V, Battistella M, Sokol H, Lemarchand N, Marteau P. Crohn's disease of the vulva. *J Crohns Colitis* 2014;8:563–70.

Foo WC, Papalas JA, Robboy SJ, Selim MA. Vulvar manifestations of Crohn's disease. *Am J Dermatopathol* 2011;33:588–93.

Girszyn N, Leport J, Arnaud L, Kahn JE, Piette AM, Bletry O. Crohn's disease affecting only vulvoperineal area. *Presse Med* 2007;36:1762–5.

Gunthert AR, Hinney B, Nesselhut K. Vulvitis granulomatosa and unilateral hypertrophy of the vulva related to Crohn's disease: A case report. *Am J Obstet Gynecol* 2004;1915:1719–20.

Leu S, Sun PK, Collyer J, Smidt A, Stika CS, Schlosser B, Mirowski GW, Vanagunas A, Buchman AL. Clinical spectrum of vulva metastatic Crohn's disease. *Dig Dis Sci* 2009;54:1565–71.

Reyes M, Borum M. Severe case of genital and perianal cutaneous Crohn's disease. *Inflamm Bowel Dis* 2009;15:1125–6.

4

Vesicles

Giuseppe Micali, Maria Rita Nasca, and Pompeo Donofrio

4.1 Vesicles

4.1.1 Herpes Simplex

Clinical aspect: Primary herpes simplex (HS) is characterized by significant morbidity, long duration, general symptoms (fever, malaise, and myalgia), and significant local pain. After an incubation period ranging from 1 to 3 weeks, multiple and often clustered vesicles of approximately 0.5–0.8 mm in diameter, surrounded by erythema and edema, appear on the labia, vaginal introitus, and perineal area (Figures 4.1.1 and 4.1.2); subsequently, blisters may erode, leaving polycyclic abrasions (Figures 4.1.3 through 4.1.5) or shallow and tender ulcers (Figures 4.1.6 and 4.1.7). Frequent cervical and urethral involvement causes vaginal and urethral discharge, dysuria, and, sometimes, urinary retention. Inguinal lymph nodes are enlarged and tender.

Definition: It is a viral, usually sexually transmitted genital disease in adults, characterized by episodic recurrences after primary infection.

Etiology: Two different causative agents, HSV1 and HSV2, are known. Genital disease occurs following sexual contact with an infected individual and is predominantly associated with HSV2, although in the last two decades a marked tendency towards an increase of HSV1 genital infection has been recorded. After primary infection, which may be asymptomatic in a significant number of cases, latent HSV settles in the sacral nerve root ganglia. Reactivation following stressful events (fever, sexual intercourse, and menses, etc.) or immune suppression may cause the onset of overt infection or asymptomatic virus shedding.

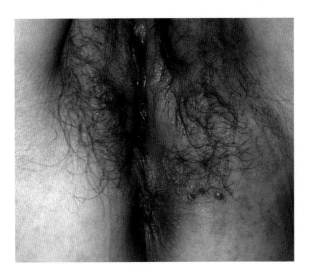

FIGURE 4.1.1   Multiple clustered blisters: herpes simplex.

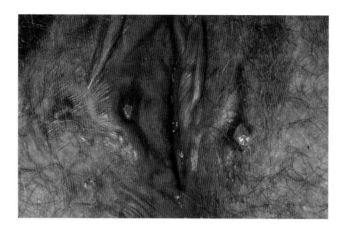

FIGURE 4.1.2   Shallow ulcers resulting from vesicle abrasion: herpes simplex.

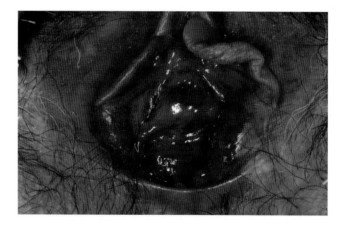

FIGURE 4.1.3   Polyciclic abrasion due to rupture of clustered herpetic blisters with surrounding erythema.

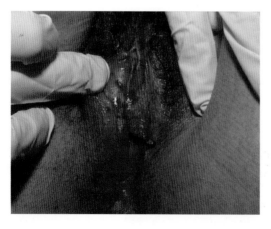

FIGURE 4.1.4   Policyclic abrasions with prominent erythema: herpes simplex.

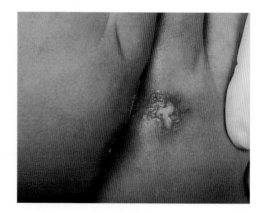

FIGURE 4.1.5   Policyclic abrasion with surrounding erythema: herpes simplex.

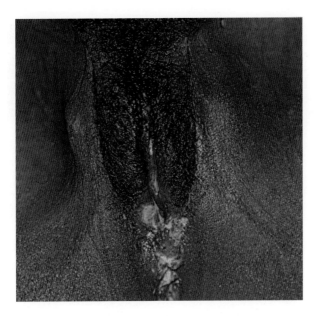

FIGURE 4.1.6 Multiple ulcerations in a dark-skinned patient: herpes simplex.

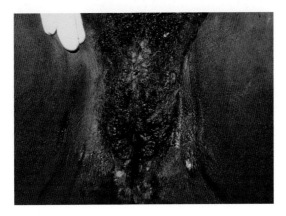

FIGURE 4.1.7 Extensive ulcerations in a dark-skinned patient: herpes simplex.

Epidemiology: It is diffused worldwide. Lifetime HSV2 seroprevalence may be as high as 80% in some series, with a recorded increase at puberty, and is higher in women than in men. However, only approximately 25% of subjects infected with HSV2 develop recurrent genital disease. Recurrence rates are lower in the case of genital infection with HSV1.

Clinical course: Recurrences are characterized by a more circumscribed eruption, preceded by less intense burning and pain, which heals in 8–10 days. HS may be associated with erythema multiforme that is recurrent after each herpes outbreak. Atypical lesions (deep long-lasting ulcers and hypertrophic lesions) may be observed in immunosuppressed individuals.

Diagnosis: Cytology smear (Tzanck test) showing the typical ballooning multinucleated giant cells may be useful, but it does not rule out herpes zoster (HZ). This may be accomplished by direct immune fluorescent techniques, which are also able to distinguish HSV1 from HSV2 infections. Alternatively, detection of HSV DNA by PCR techniques may be performed; these techniques also enable the detection of asymptomatic viral shedding. Histology may be required for atypical cases in immunosuppressed patients.

Differential diagnosis: HZ, chancroid, syphilis, aphthosis, erosive lichen planus, and fixed drug eruption.

Therapy: Treatment with antiviral nucleoside analogs (acyclovir, valacyclovir, or famciclovir) reduces morbidity, recurrences, and complications. Prevention via the use of barrier protection (condom) during sexual intercourse for subjects with a history of herpetic genital infection is essential regardless of existing lesions, as asymptomatic viral shedding may occur and cause transmission to susceptible partners.

Bibliography

Azwa A, Barton SE. Aspects of herpes simplex virus: A clinical review. *J Fam Plann Reprod Health Care* 2009;35:237–42.

Gupta R, Warren T, Wald A. Genital herpes. *Lancet* 2007;370:2127–37.

Patel R, Rompalo A. Managing patients with genital herpes and their sexual partners. *Infect Dis Clin North Am* 2005;19:427–38.

4.1.2 Herpes Zoster

Clinical aspect: The usual appearance is that of vesicles with a typical unilateral localization, involving the area of distribution of a sensitive nerve ending (dermatome) (Figures 4.1.8 and 4.1.9). Friction in intertriginous areas may easily cause abrasions consequent to blister breakdown. Distant lesions may develop in immunosuppressed patients as the result of viral dissemination.

Definition: It is due to a local recurrence of varicella zoster virus (VZV) infection and follows chickenpox after several years.

Etiology: After primary infection, the virus settles at the root of sensitive ganglia and from there spreads through the territory of innervation of a sensitive nerve in case of reactivation from a latent stage. Genital lesions may occur as the result of viral spread through the nervum pudendum.

Epidemiology: It has been reported that almost 30% of the general population develops HZ during their lifetime. Frequency increases with age, and incidence is much higher in immunosuppressed patients.

Clinical course: HZ usually breaks out with local paresthesias or pain, followed after 24–48 hours by the onset of vesicles in the involved site. General symptoms are infrequent. Lesions progress for 5–7 days and then start to heal, usually without scarring but with frequent residual hypo- or hyperpigmentation.

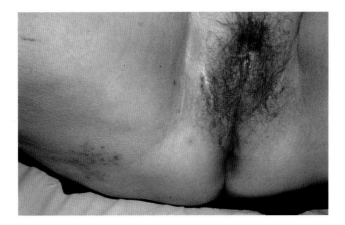

FIGURE 4.1.8   Clustered blisters extending to the right buttock: herpes zoster.

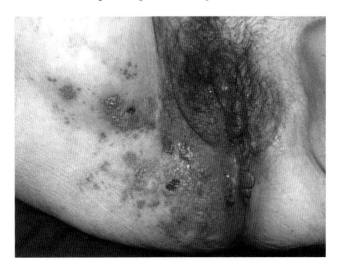

FIGURE 4.1.9   Extensive herpetiform blistering and erythema with unilateral dermatomeric distribution; ipsilateral vulvar edema is also present: herpes zoster.

Postherpetic neuralgia is a major complication, especially in the elderly. Unlike HS, HZ usually does not recur in immunocompetent patients.

Diagnosis: If the clinical features are typical, other diagnostic procedures are seldom required.

Differential diagnosis: Differential diagnosis of HZ involving the genital area includes HS infection. HZ occurs in a dermatomal unilateral distribution and is more frequent in the elderly. Chickenpox, aphthosis, cellulitis, and contact dermatitis may also be considered.

Therapy: The lesions heal spontaneously in immunocompetent patients. The aim of treatment is to speed clinical recovery and to control the associated pain. Therapy with oral acyclovir, valacyclovir, famciclovir, and brivudin has been shown to be effective on the severity and duration of HZ if initiated no longer than 48 hours after the onset of the skin rash. It has been reported that early therapy can reduce the risk of postherpetic neuralgia. For this reason, prompt treatment is recommended in patients over the age of 60 years. A vaccine has recently become available.

Bibliography

Birch CJ, Druce JD, Catton MC, MacGregor L, Read T. Detection of varicella zoster virus in genital specimens using a multiplex polymerase chain reaction. *Sex Transm Infect* 2003;79:298–300.

Brown D. Herpes zoster of the vulva. *Clin Obstet Gynecol* 1972;15:1010–4.

Dhiman N, Wright PA, Espy MJ, Schneider SK, Smith TF, Pritt BS. Concurrent detection of herpes simplex and varicella-zoster viruses by polymerase chain reaction from the same anatomic location. *Diagn Microbiol Infect Dis* 2011;70:538–40.

4.1.3 Chickenpox

Clinical aspect: It is characterized by a diffuse rash of red, itchy spots that soon turn into fluid-filled vesicles. Lesion progression occurs within 24 hours through the following five stages: (1) small spots of erythema; (2) thin-walled blisters filled with clear fluid; (3) cloudy blisters; (4) shallow abrasions; and (5) dry brown crusts. Repeated crops of new lesions keep appearing for 4–5 days, so all five stages are usually present at the same time. Rash is on all body surfaces, but it generally starts on the head and back. Genital lesions may occur (Figures 4.1.10 and 4.1.11) and may sometimes show prominent ulceration. The lesions are intensely pruritic and are accompanied by influenza symptoms (fever, headache, and myalgias).

Definition: It is a highly contagious viral disease typical of pediatric age.

Etiology: It is caused by VZV primary infection.

Epidemiology: It is more common in childhood.

Clinical course: Healing occurs after 1–2 weeks when the crusts fall off naturally. Common complications may be secondary bacterial infection and permanent scarring. Although usually self-limited, chickenpox can also sometimes cause more serious complications, including pneumonia and encephalitis.

Diagnosis: It is clinical.

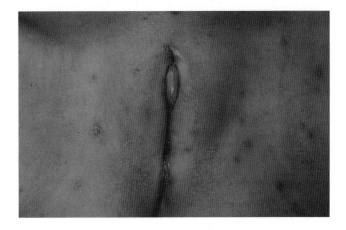

FIGURE 4.1.10 Multiple scattered vesicles filled with clear fluid: chickenpox.

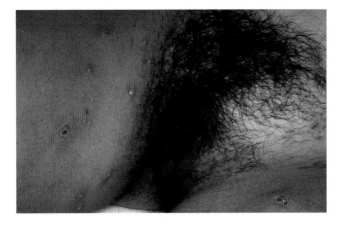

FIGURE 4.1.11 Multiple scattered vesicles and round abrasions: chickenpox.

Differential diagnosis: HS, HZ, bacterial infections (impetigo), insect bites, smallpox, syphilis, and Dühring disease.

Therapy: It is symptomatic in most cases. Systemic antivirals are recommended only in selected patients, such as immunosuppressed individuals. A vaccine is also available.

Bibliography

Simon HK, Steele DW. Varicella: Pediatric genital/rectal vesicular lesions of unclear origin. *Ann Emerg Med* 1995;25:111–4.

4.1.4 Contact Dermatitis

Clinical aspect: Contact with irritants or allergenic substances may result in the development of variably sized vesicles arising on reddened skin (Figures 4.1.12 through 4.1.14) that may easily undergo secondary infection, turning into oozing superficial abrasions. Burning and/or pruritus are common findings.

Definition: It is a skin inflammation induced by an external agent acting as an irritant (irritant CD [ICD]) or an allergen (allergic CD [ACD]). There is a spectrum from the acute stage, with mild local erythema or blistering and weeping lesions, to the chronic, late forms, with thick, fissured, and lichenified plaques.

Etiology: The inflammatory reaction is caused by physical or chemical agents acting by means of a direct nonimmunologic cytotoxic effect in the case of primary ICD or of a delayed, cell-mediated, type IV immune response in sensitized individuals in the case of ACD.

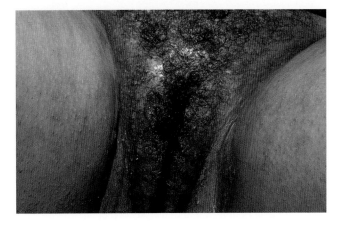

FIGURE 4.1.12 Diffuse erythema with scattered vesicles: acute contact dermatitis.

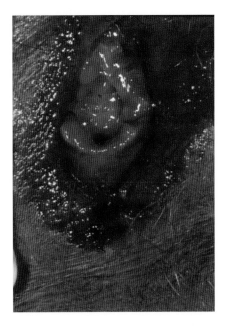

FIGURE 4.1.13 Superficial oozing abrasions resulting from blister rupture: acute contact dermatitis.

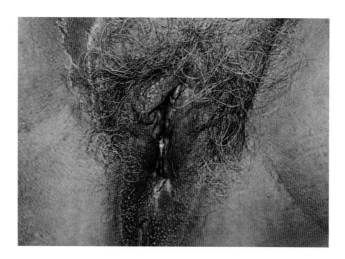

FIGURE 4.1.14 Erythema with peripheral scaling and ensuing lichenification in subacute contact dermatitis.

Epidemiology: The reported incidence of CD, either acute or chronic, ranges from 15% (Australia) to 30% (UK) in vulvar clinics.

Clinical course: If the offending agent is identified and removed, ACD and ICD subside. If not, chronicization may ensue. Bacterial or yeast superinfections frequently occur.

Diagnosis: The diagnosis of vulvar CD is usually made by taking a detailed history and by careful physical examination. Patch tests may be helpful for identifying ACD; if they are negative, and symptoms are reported to occur immediately after exposure, ICD should be considered. Biopsy may sometimes be required to rule out other conditions.

Differential diagnosis: Atopic dermatitis, candidiasis, seborrheic dermatitis, intertrigo, and bacterial infections.

Therapy: The cornerstone of treatment of CD is the identification and removal of the causative irritant or allergen. Details of the patient's daily routine for genital hygiene should be reviewed. All patients should be instructed in proper vulvar care and advised to avoid all potential irritants, including friction from tight clothes and intercourse, spermicides, and artificial lubricants, during the acute stage of the disease. Cold compresses and topical corticosteroids may be prescribed to decrease inflammation. Oral antihistamines may be used to help alleviate pruritus. Short courses of oral corticosteroids may sometimes be beneficial. Superimposed bacterial and/or fungal infections should be promptly ruled out and properly treated with antibiotics and antifungals.

Bibliography

Bauer A, Oehme S, Geier J. Contact sensitization in the anal and genital area. *Curr Probl Dermatol* 2011;40:133–41.

Beecker J. Therapeutic principles in vulvovaginal dermatology. *Dermatol Clin* 2010;28:639–48.

Burrows LJ, Shaw HA, Goldstein AT. The vulvar dermatoses. *J Sex Med* 2008;5:276–83.

Crone AM, Stewart EJ, Wojnarowska F, Powell SM. Aetiological factors in vulvar dermatitis. *J Eur Acad Dermatol Venereol* 2000;14:181–6.

Margesson LJ. Contact dermatitis of the vulva. *Dermatol Ther* 2004;17:20–7.

Vermaat H, van Meurs T, Rustemeyer T, Bruynzeel DP, Kirtschig G. Vulval allergic contact dermatitis due to peppermint oil in herbal tea. *Contact Dermatitis* 2008;58:364–5.

5

Bullae

Maria Rita Nasca and Giuseppe Micali

5.1 Bullae and/or Abrasions

5.1.1 Pemphigus Vulgaris

Clinical aspect: Typical aflegmasic flaccid and fragile bullae, soon turning to nonspecific erythematous, superficial and oozing abrasions (Figures 5.1.1 through 5.1.3), may develop on the mucosa of the inner labia and vestibule or on vulvar skin. Severe burning, soreness, and pain are constantly reported. Flaccid blisters and erosions may also occur elsewhere on distant skin or mouth.

Definition: It is an autoimmune blistering disorder affecting the skin and mucosa.

Etiology: It is caused by circulating IgG autoantibodies producing intraepithelial suprabasal acantholysis by binding to a desmosomal cadherin (desmoglein 3), a surface antigen of keratinocytes that mediates epidermal cell-to-cell adhesion.

Epidemiology: The disorder chiefly affects middle-aged to elderly adults. The incidence of pemphigus is 0.5–3.2 cases per 100,000 of the population per year. The frequency of female genital tract involvement (cervix, vagina, and vulva) is unknown, but vulvar lesions are reported in some series to occur in approximately 10% of affected patients.

Clinical course: Vulvar and/or vaginal scarring may sometimes occur in longstanding lesions. Pemphigus vulgaris (PV) is a chronic, generalized disease with a fatal outcome if left untreated. Among treated patients, complications are mostly related to the side effects of the prolonged systemic treatments.

Diagnosis: Direct immunofluorescence testing on a frozen biopsy sample obtained from perilesional skin showing intercellular deposits of IgG or C3 in the epidermis is diagnostic. Tzanck smear, indirect

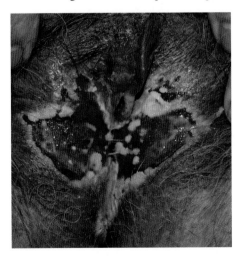

FIGURE 5.1.1 Shallow abrasions resulting from rupture of aflegmasic superficial blisters: pemphigus vulgaris.

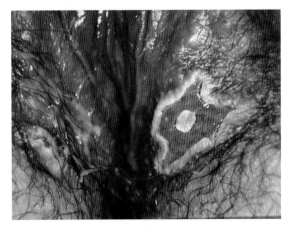

FIGURE 5.1.2 Abrasion with detached peripheral epidermis typical of pemphigus vulgaris.

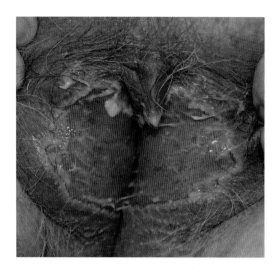

FIGURE 5.1.3   Pemphigus vulgaris.

immunofluorescence (showing circulating autoantibodies targeting desmoglein 3), immunoblotting, and enzyme-linked immunosorbent assay (ELISA) testing are also useful.

Differential diagnosis: Bullous and cicatricial pemphigoid, erosive lichen planus, fixed drug eruption, erythema multiforme, toxic epidermal necrolysis, paraneoplastic pemphigus, and Hailey–Hailey disease. When present, acantholysis in a cervicovaginal cytologic sample is known to be potentially misinterpreted as a neoplastic finding.

Therapy: PV requires lifelong treatment with systemic corticosteroids (prednisone and methylprednisolone) and/or immunosuppressants (cyclophosphamide, azathioprine, or mycophenolate mofetil). Oral antibiotics with anti-inflammatory properties (tetracycline or erythromycin), gold compounds, rituximab, plasmapheresis, and extracorporeal photochemotherapy may also be useful. Patients should be advised to follow careful local genital care in order to prevent superinfections and scarring.

Bibliography

Akhyani M, Chams-Davatchi C, Naraghi Z, Daneshpazhooh M, Toosi S, Asgari M, Malekhami F. Cervicovaginal involvement in pemphigus vulgaris: A clinical study of 77 cases. *Br J Dermatol* 2008;158:478–82.

Batta K, Munday PE, Tatnall FM. Pemphigus vulgaris localized to the vagina presenting as chronic vaginal discharge. *Br J Dermatol* 1999;140:945–7.

Fairbanks Barbosa ND, de Aguiar LM, Maruta CW, Aoki V, Sotto MN, Labinas GH, Perigo AM, Santi CG. Vulvo-cervico-vaginal manifestations and evaluation of Papanicolaou smears in pemphigus vulgaris and pemphigus foliaceus. *J Am Acad Dermatol* 2012;67:409–16.

Malik M, Ahmed AR. Involvement of the female genital tract in pemphigus vulgaris. *Obstet Gynecol* 2005;106:1005–12.

Onuma K, Kanbour-Shakir A, Modery J, Kanbour A. Pemphigus vulgaris of the vagina—Its cytomorphologic features on liquid-based cytology and pitfalls: Case report and cytological differential diagnosis. *Diagn Cytopathol* 2009;37:832–5.

Yeh SW, Sami N, Ahmed RA. Treatment of pemphigus vulgaris: Current and emerging options. *Am J Clin Dermatol* 2005;6:327–42.

5.1.2 Pemphigus Vegetans

Clinical aspect: Relatively circumscribed lesions, almost confined to the great skin fold areas, appear as dusky, papillated, vegetating, cauliflower-like, verrucous, and oozing plaques arising on abrasions corresponding to the floor of eroded bullae (Figures 5.1.4 and 5.1.5). The scalp, face, and oral mucosa, notably the labial commissures, may also be involved.

Definition: It is an unusual variant of PV, characterized by a distinctive clinical presentation, course, and response to treatment.

Etiology: Autoimmune, characterized by acantholysis due to autoantibodies targeting desmoglein 3.

Epidemiology: It accounts for 2%–7% of the cases of pemphigus.

Clinical course: Unlike PV, it has a relatively benign course.

Diagnosis: It is often challenging, as no clinical resemblance to a vesiculobullous disorder may be evident. Histopathology, supported by direct and indirect immunofluorescence, immunoblotting, and/or ELISA testing, helps with obtaining the correct diagnosis.

Differential diagnosis: Pyodermatitis vegetans associated with ulcerative colitis, pemphigoid vegetans, and acantholytic dyskeratosis.

Therapy: Systemic corticosteroids and immunosuppressive agents are usually effective at lower dosages compared with classic PV.

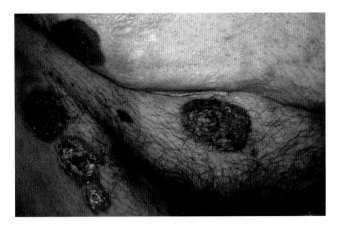

FIGURE 5.1.4   Circumscribed flaccid bullae heralding the development of raised vegetations in pemphigus vegetans.

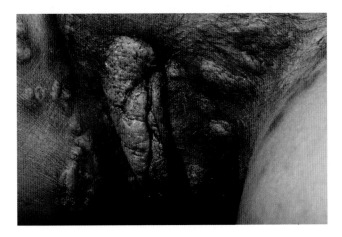

FIGURE 5.1.5   Prominent verrucous plaques replacing the blisters that in pemphigus vegetans are, with time, no longer appreciable.

Bibliography

Wong KT, Wong KK. A case of acantholytic dermatosis of the vulva with features of pemphigus vegetans. *J Cutan Pathol* 1994;21:453–6.

Zaraa I, Sellami A, Bouguerra C, Sellami MK, Chelly I, Zitouna M, Makni S, Hmida AB, Mokni M, Osman AB. Pemphigus vegetans: A clinical, histological, immunopathological and prognostic study. *J Eur Acad Dermatol Venereol* 2011;25:1160–7.

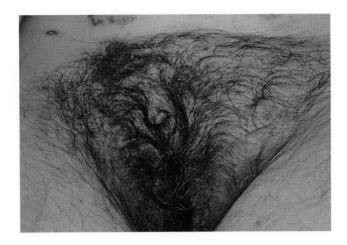

FIGURE 5.1.6 Red-yellowish scaling patches resulting from rupture of superficial flaccid bullae in pemphigus erythematosus.

5.1.3 Pemphigus Erythematosus

Clinical aspect: It represents a superficial variety of pemphigus, with the formation of small flaccid bullae, oozing superficial abrasions, scaling and crusting developing on seborrheic areas (scalp, face, upper chest, and back). Superficial blisters may also affect the vulvar skin as red–yellowish scaling patches (Figure 5.1.6). Mucous membranes are always spared.

Definition: It is an autoimmune blistering disorder affecting the skin, also known as Senear–Usher syndrome.

Etiology: It is caused by circulating autoantibodies directed towards a desmosomal cadherin (desmoglein 1) mostly expressed on the desmosomes of outer epidermal layers. Certain HLA haplotypes (A10 or A26, DRW6) are thought to be associated, suggesting a genetic predisposition.

Epidemiology: Patients with this clinical variant comprise only a small subgroup of those with pemphigus.

Clinical course: Onset and progression are typically slow. Rarely, extensive involvement may lead to exfoliative erythroderma.

Diagnosis: Direct and indirect immunofluorescence, immunoblotting and/or ELISA testing are essential for diagnosis.

Differential diagnosis: Occasionally, the appearance may suggest a papulosquamous disorder. Seborrheic dermatitis, lupus erythematosus (acute, discoid, and subacute cutaneous), atopic dermatitis, and foliaceus or paraneoplastic pemphigus should be ruled out. Impetigo, glucagonoma syndrome, and subcorneal pustular dermatosis are other possible differential diagnoses.

Therapy: Systemic steroids are the mainstay of therapy. Other useful drugs include immunosuppressive agents (azathioprine, cyclophosphamide, methotrexate, and mycophenolate mofetil), dapsone, tetracycline, niacinamide, and hydroxychloroquine.

Bibliography

Braunstein I, Werth V. Treatment of dermatologic connective tissue disease and autoimmune blistering disorders in pregnancy. *Dermatol Ther* 2013;26:354–63.

Ruocco E, Wolf R, Ruocco V, Brunetti G, Romano F, Lo Schiavo A. Pemphigus: Associations and management guidelines: Facts and controversies. *Clin Dermatol* 2013;31:382–90.

Vassileva S, Drenovska K, Manuelyan K. Autoimmune blistering dermatoses as systemic diseases. *Clin Dermatol* 2014;32:364–75.

5.1.4 Bullous Pemphigoid

Clinical aspect: Vulvar lesions are uncommon and more often occur as part of a generalized eruption extending to the skin of the pubic area, the lower abdomen, and the inner aspect of the thighs. They appear as tense vesicles and large bullae (up to 5 cm in diameter), typically arising within sharply defined patches of erythema (Figures 5.1.7 and 5.1.8), which soon result in shallow abrasions following mild mechanical traumas. Local irritation and intense pruritus, which can be generalized, are common complaints.

Definition: It is an uncommon cutaneous autoimmune blistering disorder.

Etiology: It is due to circulating IgG autoantibodies directed towards two different hemidesmosomal antigens of 230 and 180 kDa (BPAG1 and BPAG2) located in the basement membrane zone, with consequent inflammation and subepidermal splitting.

Epidemiology: It is rare. Onset is usually after 60 years of age.

Clinical course: Genital erosions usually heal without permanent scarring and show a relatively mild and benign, although chronic, course.

Diagnosis: The presence of typical lesions in other skin areas is usually useful for determining the diagnosis, which is made based on the detection of linear deposits of IgG and/or C3 at the basal membrane zone on immunofluorescent histopathology. Circulating antibasement membrane antibodies are present in 70% of cases.

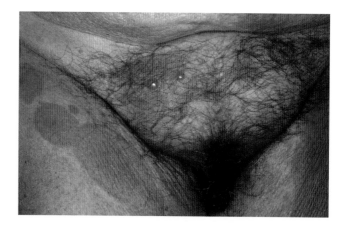

FIGURE 5.1.7   Tense bullae arising within areas of patchy erythema in bullous pemphigoid.

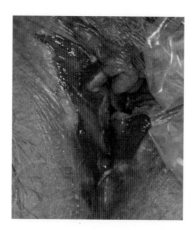

FIGURE 5.1.8   Shallow abrasions resulting from the rupture of blisters in bullous pemphigoid.

Differential diagnosis: PV, bullous fixed drug eruptions, cicatricial pemphigoid, Dühring disease, erythema multiforme, erosive lichen planus, epidermolysis bullosa, and lichen sclerosus (scarring).

Therapy: Systemic and topical steroids are the mainstay of treatment. Other immunosuppressive agents, such as azathioprine, cyclophosphamide, methotrexate, and mycophenolate mofetil, can be used in resistant cases. Dapsone and other oral agents with anti-inflammatory effects, such as tetracycline or macrolides (erythromycin), may be used in mild or localized disease.

Bibliography

Atzori L, Pau M, Podda R, Manieli C, Aste N. A case of bullous pemphigoid in infancy treated with local corticosteroids. *G Ital Dermatol Venereol* 2011;146:493–6.

Farrell AM, Kirtschig G, Dalziel KL, Allen J, Dootson G, Edwards S, Wojnarowska F. Childhood vulval pemphigoid: A clinical and immunopathological study of five patients. *Br J Dermatol* 1999;140:308–12.

Fischer G, Rogers M. Vulvar disease in children: A clinical audit of 130 cases. *Pediatr Dermatol* 2000;17:1–6.

Fisler RE, Saeb M, Liang MG, Howard RM, McKee PH. Childhood bullous pemphigoid: A clinicopathologic study and review of the literature. *Am J Dermatopathol* 2003;25:183–9.

Hertl M, Niedermeier A, Borradori L. Autoimmune bullous skin disorders. *Ther Umsch* 2010;67:465–82.

Ingen-Housz-Oro S, Valeyrie-Allanore L, Ortonne N, Roujeau JC, Wolkenstein P, Chosidow O. Management of bullous pemphigoid with topical steroids in the clinical practice of a single center: Outcome at 6 and 12 months. *Dermatology* 2011;222:176–9.

Urano S. Localized bullous pemphigoid of the vulva. *J Dermatol* 1996;23:580–2.

5.1.5 Benign Familial Pemphigus (Hailey–Hailey Disease)

Clinical aspect: Lesions typically occur on the neck, axillae, inguinal folds, and anogenital area. Crops of vesicles and bullae, often surrounded by erythema, easily erode and develop abrasions with crusting or superimposed infections and usually develop in the groin, extending to the neighboring areas of the inner thighs and vulva (Figures 5.1.9 and 5.1.10), down along the edges of the labia majora. Deep fissures in the inguinal crease may be observed, whereas mucosal involvement is rare. Local discomfort, burning, itching, and pain are often reported.

Definition: It is a rare autosomal dominant superficial blistering disease of the intertriginous areas.

Etiology: It is an acantholytic disorder due to an intrinsic desmosomal fragility, resulting from a mutation of the *ATP2C1* gene on band 3q21–q24, which encodes the calcium pump protein Ca^{2+}-ATPase. Recurrent blistering eruptions are usually precipitated by environmental triggering factors (e.g., increased temperature and humidity, mechanical or chemical irritants, and infections).

Epidemiology: It is a rare condition that is diffused worldwide, with a prevalence of approximately 1/50,000. Onset of symptoms may be delayed until 30–49 years of age.

Clinical course: A foul-smelling drainage occurs in some cases as a result of secondary infection. A history of multiple relapses and remissions is characteristic. The symptoms worsen during summer, when the rises in environmental temperature and humidity facilitate superinfections in the intertriginous areas.

Diagnosis: It is usually suggested by clinical features and family history. A skin biopsy showing characteristic histology with layers of acantholytic detached skin cells ("dilapidated brick wall") readily confirms the diagnosis. Unlike PV, immunofluorescence testing is negative.

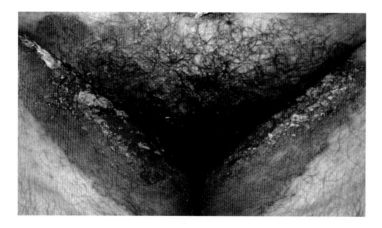

FIGURE 5.1.9   Blistering and erosions predominantly involving the inguinal creases in Hailey–Hailey disease.

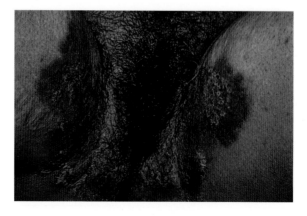

FIGURE 5.1.10   Blistering and crusting in Hailey–Hailey disease.

Differential diagnosis: Intertrigo, bacterial and fungal infections (including erythrasma and dermatophytosis), autoimmune blistering disorders (PV and cicatricial pemphigoid), bullous fixed drug eruption, erythema multiforme, herpes simplex, extramammary Paget disease, and psoriasis.

Therapy: Therapeutic options are limited. Treatment is aimed at the control of local environmental precipitating factors and superinfections. Soothing compresses followed by intermittent use of low-to-mid-potency corticosteroids and topical antibiotics (usually erythromycin or clindamycin) result in transient improvements. Bacterial culture and sensitivity can help guide appropriate therapy. In refractory patients, systemic treatments, such as dapsone, corticosteroids, methotrexate, and retinoids (isotretinoin or acitretin), may be attempted with some success. Anecdotal improvements with narrow-band ultraviolet B phototherapy have recently been reported.

Bibliography

Leinonen PT, Hagg PM, Peltonen S, Jouhilahti EM, Melkko J, Korkiamäki T, Oikarinen A, Peltonen J. Reevaluation of the normal epidermal calcium gradient, and analysis of calcium levels and ATP receptors in Hailey–Hailey and Darier epidermis. *J Invest Dermatol* 2009;129:1379–87.

Nasca MR, De Pasquale R, Amodeo S, Micali G. Treatment of Hailey–Hailey diseases with oral erythromycin. *J Dermatol Treatment* 2000;11:273–7.

Vilmer C, Dehen L. Condylomatous vulvar form of Hailey–Hailey's disease. *Ann Dermatol Venereol* 2004;131:607–8.

Wieselthier JS, Pincus SH. Hailey–Hailey disease of the vulva. *Arch Dermatol* 1993;129:1344–5.

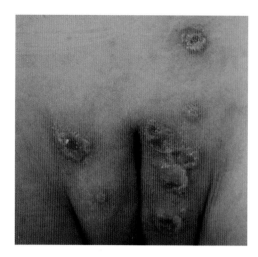

FIGURE 5.2.1   Clustered crops of blisters: linear IgA bullous dermatitis.

5.2 Bullae and/or Abrasions plus Scarring

5.2.1 Linear IgA Bullous Dermatitis

Clinical aspect: It is characterized by tense bullae and abrasions located in the genital region (Figure 5.2.1) and later affecting the hands, feet, and face, with lesions typically arranged in a "cluster of jewels-like" pattern. Some patients report a prolonged period of prodromal itching or transient pruritus or burning before lesions appear.

Definition: Linear IgA bullous disease is an autoimmune subepidermal blistering disorder associated with autoantibodies directed against the transmembrane hemidesmosomal protein BP180/type XVII collagen.

Etiology: It may be idiopathic or drug induced (vancomycin).

Epidemiology: It is generally a childhood disorder that occurs before puberty, although it may also be observed in the elderly.

Clinical course: The lesions may appear abruptly or be chronically relapsing and may cause scarring when involving mucosal sites, mimicking cicatricial pemphigoid.

Diagnosis: Reviews of medication exposures and delineations of the drug time line are crucial for identifying potential inciting agents. The diagnosis is confirmed by immunofluorescence microscopy. Serum should be obtained for indirect immunofluorescence studies and ELISA testing. Approximately 50% of patients with linear IgA dermatosis have detectable circulating antibodies that bind to the basal membrane zone.

Differential diagnosis: Epidermolysis bullosa, cicatricial pemphigoid, Dühring disease, and bacterial infection (impetigo).

Therapy: A medical treatment may be run with topical corticosteroids and oral dapsone.

Bibliography

Kenani N, Mebazaa A, Denguezli M, Ghariani N, Sriha B, Belajouza C, Nouira R. Childhood linear IgA bullous dermatosis in Tunisia. *Pediatr Dermatol* 2009;26:28–33.

Kharfi M, Khaled A, Karaa A, Zaraa I, Fazaa B, Kamoun MR. Linear IgA bullous dermatosis: The more frequent bullous dermatosis of children. *Dermatol Online J* 2010;16:2.

Kneisel A, Hertl M. Autoimmune bullous skin diseases. Part 1: Clinical manifestations. *J Dtsch Dermatol Ges* 2011;9:844–56.

Legrain V, Taieb A, Surlève-Bazeille JE, Bernard P, Maleville J. Linear IgA dermatosis of childhood: Case report with an immunoelectron microscopic study. *Pediatr Dermatol* 1991;8:310–3.

5.2.2 Erythema Multiforme

Clinical aspect: Vulvar skin and mucosal involvement is frequent in erythema multiforme major. Symmetrical patches of erythema may show a typical iris pattern and eventually progress to the development of extensive bullae, which may cause the formation of abrasions (Figure 5.2.2), with consequent scarring in later stages. Widespread flaccid bullous blistering may result in massive skin and mucosal sheet-like detachment with dermal denudation (toxic epidermal necrolysis). Vaginal involvement results in a desquamative vaginitis with purulent discharge. Pain, burning, and dysuria are prominent. Mouth, eyes, and distal extremities can present a symmetric vesiculobullous eruption. These patients are acutely ill, with fever, malaise, and myalgias.

Definition: It is an acute inflammatory mucocutaneous disorder resulting from a hypersensitivity reaction usually triggered by infections or drugs.

Etiology: Common infections, such as HSV or *Streptococcus*, and some drugs, such as sulfonamides, antibiotics (penicillin), nonsteroidal anti-inflammatory drugs, phenytoin, carbamazepine, and barbiturates, are recognized as possible causative agents. In approximately 50% of cases, the etiology is unknown.

Epidemiology: Globally, its frequency is estimated at approximately 1.2–6 cases per million individuals per year.

Clinical course: Lesions are usually self-limited and heal spontaneously with hyper- and/or hypopigmentation in 1–2 weeks. Recurrences are common following recurrent HSV infection or with repeated drug exposure. The major variant has a more protracted course (3–6 weeks) and a mortality rate (<5%) related to loss of the cutaneous barrier and secondary sepsis, which is directly proportional to the involved total body surface area.

Diagnosis: Diagnosis is mainly based on patient history and clinical observation. Careful inspection of other skin areas, as well as of the oral mucosa, is recommended. A skin biopsy is mandatory to confirm the diagnosis.

Differential diagnosis: PV, bullous pemphigoid, linear IgA bullous dermatitis, fixed drug eruption, toxic epidermal necrolysis, and erosive lichen planus.

Therapy: Identification and withdrawal of precipitating factors, such as drug discontinuation and treatment of underlying infections, are essential in order to obtain recovery. The use of systemic corticosteroid therapy is controversial. Most severe and extensive cases are best managed in a hospital in a burn unit.

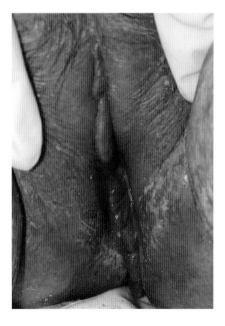

FIGURE 5.2.2 Extensive abrasions with reddening in erythema multiforme major.

Bibliography

Meneux E, Wolkenstein P, Haddad B, Roujeau JC, Revuz J, Paniel BJ. Vulvovaginal involvement in toxic epidermal necrolysis: A retrospective study of 40 cases. *Obstet Gynecol* 1998;91:283–7.

Piérard GE, Paquet P. Facing up to toxic epidermal necrolysis. *Expert Opin Pharmacother* 2010;11:2443–6.

Sokumbi O, Wetter DA. Clinical features, diagnosis, and treatment of erythema multiforme: A review for the practicing dermatologist. *Int J Dermatol* 2012;51:889–902.

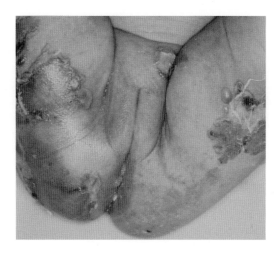

FIGURE 5.2.3 Relapsing bullae from trivial traumas due to increased skin fragility in congenital dystrophic epidermolysis bullosa.

5.2.3 Epidermolysis Bullosa

Clinical aspect: Mucous membranes, including those of the genitalia, may be involved with bullae and abrasions (Figure 5.2.3).

Definition: Group of congenital inherited disorders characterized by skin fragility.

Etiology: These diseases are due to a genetic defect in the epidermal, junctional, or dermal components underlying the physiological mechanical properties of the skin.

Epidemiology: Congenital blistering diseases are rare, but vulval involvement is common across the spectrum of these disorders.

Clinical course: Long-term prognosis is good for superficial blistering. In the dystrophic variants of this disorder, disabling scarring and adhesions, with consequent vaginal obstruction and obstructive uropathy, may occur.

Diagnosis: Biopsy for histopathologic examination and genetic investigations to identify the mutated gene are required.

Differential diagnosis: Friction blisters, autoimmune bullous disorders (bullous pemphigoid, cicatricial pemphigoid, PV, and epidermolysis bullosa acquisita), bullous fixed drug eruptions, erythema multiforme, erosive lichen planus, bacterial infections (impetigo), and staphylococcal scalded skin syndrome.

Therapy: It is challenging. It requires proper wound care, trauma avoidance, and the prevention and treatment of superinfections. Future goals are represented by protein and gene therapies.

Bibliography

Holbrook KA. Extracutaneous epithelial involvement in inherited epidermolysis bullosa. *Arch Dermatol* 1988;124:726–31.

Lataifeh I, Barahmeh S, Amarin Z, Jaradat I. Stage III squamous cell carcinoma of the vulva with groin nodes metastasis in a patient with epidermolysis bullosa. *J Obstet Gynaecol* 2010;30:750–2.

Leverkus M, Ambach A, Hoefeld-Fegeler M, Kohlhase J, Schmidt E, Schumann H, Has C, Gollnick H. Late-onset inversa recessive dystrophic epidermolysis bullosa caused by glycine substitutions in collagen type VII. *Br J Dermatol* 2011;164:1104–6.

Petersen CS, Brocks K, Weismann K, Kobayasi T, Thomsen HK. Pretibial epidermolysis bullosa with vulvar involvement. *Acta Derm Venereol* 1996;76:80–1.

Shackelford GD, Bauer EA, Graviss ER, McAlister WH. Upper airway and external genital involvement in epidermolysis bullosa dystrophica. *Radiology* 1982;143:429–32.

6

Pustules/Abscess

Giuseppe Micali, Nella Pulvirenti, and Stefano Veraldi

6.1 Pustules/Abscess

6.1.1 Fungal/Bacterial Infection

Clinical aspect: Multiple yellowish to white pustules surrounded by erythema may be observed in bacterial and candidal vulvovaginitis, respectively. Yeast infections are characterized by tiny multiple elements scattered throughout the involved areas (Figures 6.1.1 through 6.1.3). Bacterial infections frequently involve the follicular openings when the hair-bearing vulvar skin is implicated (folliculitis) (Figure 6.1.4). Pruritus and burning are commonly reported symptoms.

Definition: It is an acute vulvovaginal inflammation caused by bacteria and/or yeasts.

Etiology: Sporadic nonvenereal vulvovaginal infections may be caused either by common anaerobic and aerobic bacteria (*Staphylococcus* or *Streptococcus*), *Candida* sp., or both. Risk factors include local (irritation, occlusion, and maceration) and systemic conditions (diabetes and immune suppression).

Epidemiology: These are frequent, underreported conditions whose precise incidence is difficult to establish.

Diagnosis: A swab for bacterial/fungal culture is the most effective tool for determining the correct diagnosis.

Clinical course: Bacterial infection may be complicated by fever and abscess formation, whereas untreated yeast infection more often evolves into chronic candidiasis.

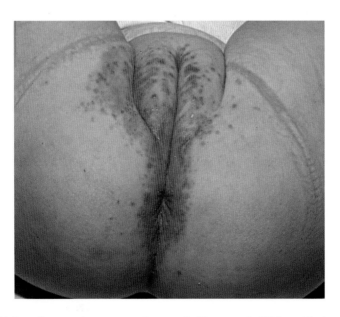

FIGURE 6.1.1 Multiple confluent erythematous papules topped with scattered whitish pustules in candidiasis.

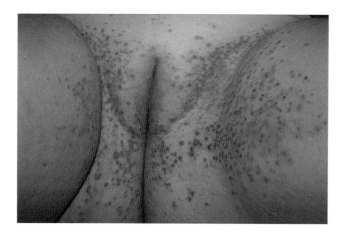

FIGURE 6.1.2   Candidiasis: typical presentation.

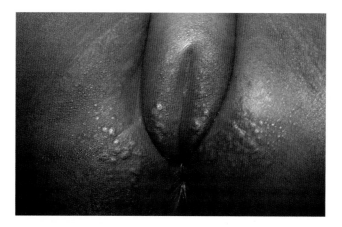

FIGURE 6.1.3   Candidiasis in a dark-skinned patient.

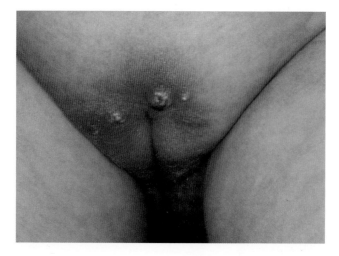

FIGURE 6.1.4   Bacterial folliculitis resulting in diffuse erythema with superimposed scattered yellowish pustules: bacterial infection.

Differential diagnosis: Hidradenitis suppurativa, chancroid, Crohn's disease, subcorneal pustular dermatosis, pustular psoriasis, amicrobic pustulosis of the folds.

Therapy: Topical and/or systemic treatment with antibiotics and/or antifungals are indicated, as suggested by microbiological investigations.

Bibliography

Hamad M, Kazandji N, Awadallah S, Allam H. Prevalence and epidemiological characteristics of vaginal candidiasis in the UAE. *Mycoses* 2014;57:184–90.

Heymann WR. Streptococcal vulvovaginitis. *J Am Acad Dermatol* 2009;61:94–5.

Mirowski GW, Schlosser BJ, Stika CS. Cutaneous vulvar streptococcal infection. *J Low Genit Tract Dis* 2012;16:281–4.

6.1.2 Folliculitis

Clinical aspect: Isolated or scattered follicular pustules, usually surrounded by an erythematous halo, may be observed in the hair-bearing areas of the vulva (Figures 6.1.5 and 6.1.6).

Definition: It is an inflammation of the vulva due to an infection of the pubic hair follicles.

Etiology: It is more often caused by *Staphylococcus aureus*, although other microorganisms (including Gram-negative bacteria, such as *Pseudomonas aeruginosa*, and fungi, such as *Candida albicans*) may occasionally be detected.

Epidemiology: It is considered to be a common disorder, although its prevalence in the genital area is unknown.

Clinical course: In the late stages of the infection, crusted lesions may be seen.

Diagnosis: Diagnosis is based on Gram staining and microbiological culture, which confirm the infection and identify the causative agent.

Differential diagnosis: Hidradenitis suppurativa, fungal infections (candidiasis and dermatophytosis), and amicrobial pustulosis of the folds.

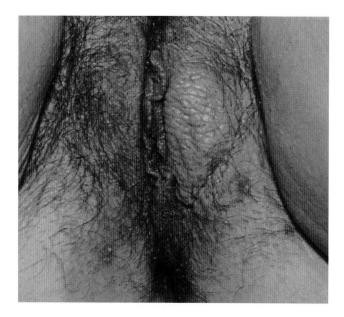

FIGURE 6.1.5   Scattered follicular pustules in folliculitis.

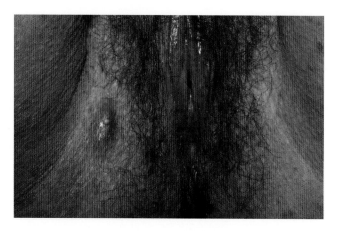

FIGURE 6.1.6   Erythematous pustule with yellowish discharge: folliculitis.

Therapy: Keeping the area clean and dry may be sufficient, since the lesions generally heal spontaneously. If the infection is more severe or recurrent, topical antibiotics and antiseptics are recommended.

Bibliography

Fischer G, Rogers M. Vulvar disease in children: A clinical audit of 130 cases. *Pediatr Dermatol* 2000;17:1–6.

Nyirjesy P, Nixon JM, Jordan CA, Buckley HR. *Malassezia furfur* folliculitis of the vulva: Olive oil solves the mystery. *Obstet Gynecol* 1994;84:710–1.

Singh N, Thappa DM, Jaisankar TJ, Habeebullah S. Pattern of non-venereal dermatoses of female external genitalia in South India. *Dermatol Online J* 2008;14:1.

6.2 Pustules/Abscess plus Scarring

6.2.1 Hidradenitis Suppurativa

Clinical aspect: It occurs in the apocrine gland-bearing areas of the armpits, groin, perianal, perineal, and gluteal regions, but the scalp may also be involved (dissecting folliculitis). In the vulva and pubic area, multiple and confluent erythematous acneiform pustules, papules, and scattered comedones may be evident; the labia and clitoris may also be affected (Figures 6.2.1 through 6.2.3). Less severe cases may only present as a cluster of two or three blackheads that communicate under the skin. However, a common finding is extensive and deep chronic inflammation, leading to subcutaneous nodules and cysts that may ulcerate and coalesce to form conglobate plaques, with underlying abscesses and draining sinuses that heal incompletely, causing extensive cord-like scarring. Oozing nodules with purulent yellow discharge are usually very painful.

Definition: Chronic suppurative inflammatory disorder in areas rich of apocrine glands, also known as Verneuil's disease or acne inversa.

Etiology: The cause is unknown. Bacterial infection has been thought to occur secondarily, following an as-yet unidentified primary defect of the follicular epithelium. Predisposing conditions include

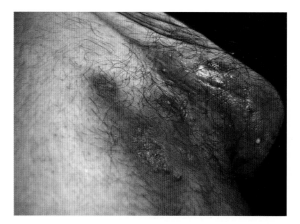

FIGURE 6.2.1 Conglobate plaques with draining sinuses and cord-like scarring: hidradenitis suppurativa.

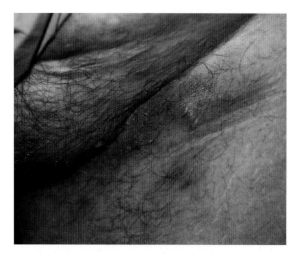

FIGURE 6.2.2 Conglobate erythematous plaques with oozing nodules and yellow purulent discharge: hidradenitis suppurativa.

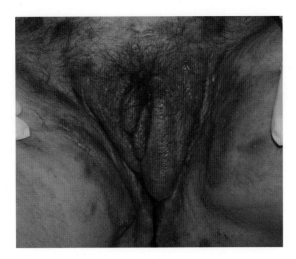

FIGURE 6.2.3 Persistent indurated edema resulting from chronic inflammation: hidradenitis suppurativa.

a positive family history, hyperandrogenism, obesity, and environmental factors, such as occlusion and maceration due to heat, humidity, and friction from clothing, chemical irritants, smoking, and lithium exposure.

Epidemiology: Its exact incidence is unknown. Women are more likely than men to develop hidradenitis suppurativa. People who have a history of acne have a higher risk of developing this condition. Hidradenitis suppurativa may run in families.

Clinical course: Once the disease begins, it grows progressively worse. Early in the disease, pustular flares occur cyclically, because the secretory activity of the apocrine glands corresponds to the progestational phase of the menstrual cycle. As the disease relentlessly progresses, the entire anogenital area becomes honeycombed and inflamed, with recurrent underlying infection. This disabling condition can cause considerable discomfort to patients, hamper movements of the affected areas, and significantly impair the quality of life. Scarring is also a common cause of significant cosmetic concerns. Other potential complications include dermal contractions, local or disseminated infections, and lymphedema caused by lymphatic injury from inflammation and arthritis.

Diagnosis: There are no specific diagnostic tests available. The diagnosis is usually based on the typical signs and symptoms.

Differential diagnosis: Bacterial/fungal infections, erysipelas, Crohn's disease, pyoderma gangrenosum, lymphogranuloma venereum, and granuloma inguinale.

Therapy: Treatment is difficult and often inadequate. In the early and mild stages, topical antiseptic cleansers and antibiotics may be useful for reducing bacterial load. In moderate-to-severe cases, systemic antibiotics (erythromycin, tetracycline, minocycline, and doxycycline) and isotretinoin should be prescribed. Treatment with biologic agents has been attempted. Severe hidradenitis may require steroid injections, surgical drainage and, sometimes, surgical removal of the affected skin areas.

Bibliography

Alharbi Z, Kauczok J, Pallua N. A review of wide surgical excision of hidradenitis suppurativa. *BMC Dermatol* 2012;12:9.

Alikhan A, Lynch PJ, Eisen DB. Hidradenitis suppurativa: A comprehensive review. *J Am Acad Dermatol* 2009;60:539–61.

Brown CF, Gallup DG, Brown VM. Hidradenitis suppurativa of the anogenital region: Response to isotretinoin. *Am J Obstet Gynecol* 1988;158:12–5.

Collier F, Smith RC, Morton CA. Diagnosis and management of hidradenitis suppurativa. *BMJ* 2013;346:f2121.

Scheinfeld N. Hidradenitis suppurativa: A practical review of possible medical treatments based on over 350 hidradenitis patients. *Dermatol Online J* 2013;19:1.

7

Papules

Maria Rita Nasca, Federica Dall'Oglio, and Giuseppe Micali

7.1 Papules

7.1.1 Molluscum Contagiosum

Clinical aspect: The lesions may be observed on the vulvar skin, the pubis, the lower abdomen, the perineum, and the buttocks. They are often multiple, of a few millimeters in diameter and appear as skin-colored or waxy, smooth, rounded, dome-shaped papules with a typical central depression containing a keratotic plug that may be easily expressed using forceps (Figures 7.1.1 through 7.1.3). Sometimes, giant

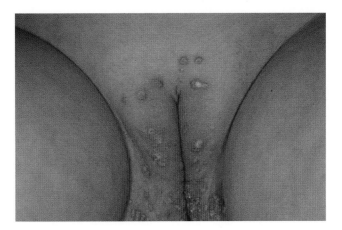

FIGURE 7.1.1   Dome-shaped papules with prominent central depression: molluscum contagiosum.

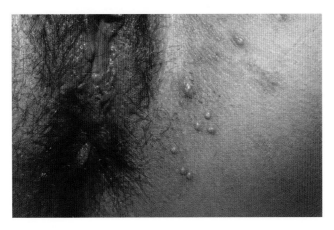

FIGURE 7.1.2   Multiple skin-colored, smooth and waxy papules: molluscum contagiosum.

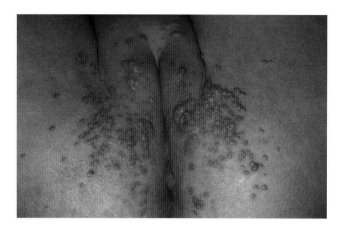

FIGURE 7.1.3   Extensive vulvo-perineal involvement in long-standing molluscum contagiosum.

lesions reaching 1 or 2 cm in diameter may be observed. They are asymptomatic, but may occasionally cause irritation and be surrounded by an area of erythema.

Definition: It is a viral infection that may affect the genital and perigenital areas of sexually active adults.

Etiology: The causative agent is a DNA poxvirus.

Epidemiology: It shows no sex predilection and its incidence is not reliably known. It is a relatively common sexually transmitted disease, although transmission from nonsexual contact (swimming pools and gym equipment, etc.), with typical lesions mostly located on the upper body, often occurs, especially in children.

Clinical course: The course is benign, and self-healing may occur over approximately 18 months or more, sometimes leaving a slightly depressed scar. On the other hand, relapses after removal are common (35% of cases).

Diagnosis: The clinical features are usually diagnostic. A typical pattern that is recognizable at dermatoscopy is a central white to yellow polylobular amorphous structure surrounded by reddish, linear or branched vessels that do not cross the midline of the lesion (Figure 7.1.4). Histology may rule out atypical cases.

Differential diagnosis: In patients with AIDS, giant lesions may resemble cryptococcosis, histoplasmosis, coccidioidomycosis, or aspergillosis. Similar clinical features may sometimes be shared by warts, epidermal cysts (milia), sebaceous hyperplasias, foreign body granulomas, keratoacanthomas, eccrine poromas, perforating disorders, and nodular basal cell carcinomas.

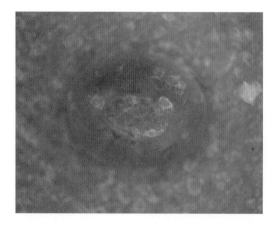

FIGURE 7.1.4   Dermoscopy of molluscum contagiosum: presence of central polyglobular white-yellowish amorphous structure with a surrounding peripheral crown of vessels.

Therapy: Surgical ablation by curettage is effective. Follow-up is recommended to promptly treat any relapse and prevent further spreading. Patients should be instructed to avoid close contact and clothes or towel sharing.

Bibliography

Castronovo C, Lebas E, Nikkels-Tassoudji N, Nikkels AF. Viral infections of the pubis. *Int J STD AIDS* 2012;23:48–50.

Lin HY, Linn G, Liu CB, Chen CJ, Yu KJ. An immunocompromised woman with severe molluscum contagiosum that responded well to topical imiquimod: A case report and literature review. *J Low Genit Tract Dis* 2010;14:134–5.

Van Onselen J. Skin infections in children. *J Fam Health Care* 2014;24:22–4.

7.1.2 Papillomatosis

Clinical aspect: It presents with multiple and symmetrically distributed, tiny (1–3 mm), raised, elongated, fleshy, skin-colored, soft, papillary, asymptomatic papules, often arranged in rows on the inner labia minora and vestibular mucosa distal to the hymenal ring (Figures 7.1.5 through 7.1.8).

Definition: Physiologic condition representing a normal variant of the female anatomy and the equivalent of male pearly penile papules.

Etiology: The etiology of these benign fibrovascular proliferations is unknown, but is unrelated to human papillomavirus (HPV) infection.

Epidemiology: No precise epidemiological data are available, and the prevalence of papillomatosis in the general population is unknown.

Clinical course: It is uneventful.

Diagnosis: It is clinical and may be aided by noninvasive dermoscopy, showing multiple whitish–pink cobblestone or grape-like structures arranged in a few regular rows; at higher magnifications, dotted or comma-like vessels may be detected in the center of each papule.

Differential diagnosis: Anogenital warts.

Therapy: Treatment is unnecessary.

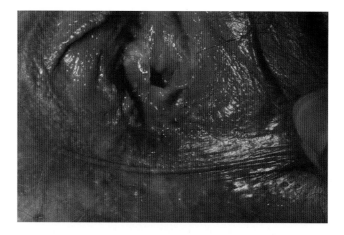

FIGURE 7.1.5 Multiple raised tiny fleshy papules: papillomatosis.

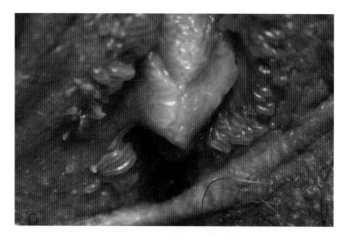

FIGURE 7.1.6 Bilateral symmetrical involvement in vulvar papillomatosis.

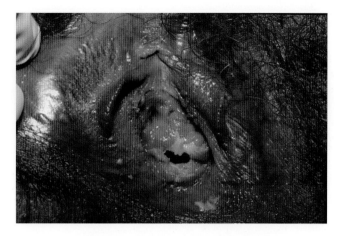

FIGURE 7.1.7   Multiple regular and symmetrically distributed elongated papules lining the vaginal opening due to vulvar papillomatosis; Fordyce spots are also appreciable in the right interlabial fold (see Section 7.1.3).

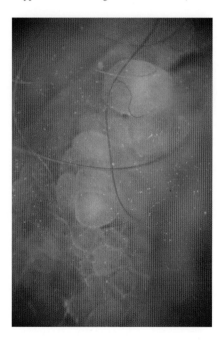

FIGURE 7.1.8   Dermoscopy of papillomatosis: presence of pinkish regular papillomatous projections.

Bibliography

Diaz Gonzales JM, Martinez Luna E, Pena Romero A, Molina Hernandez A, Dominguez Cherit J. Vestibular papillomatosis as a normal vulvar anatomical condition. *Dermatol Online J* 2013;19:20032.
Wollina U, Verma S. Vulvar vestibular papillomatosis. *Indian J Dermatol Venereol Leprol* 2010;76:270–2.

7.1.3 Sebaceous Hyperplasia/Fordyce Spots

Clinical aspect: Fordyce spots are detectable as usually multiple, small (1–3 mm), superficial, dome-shaped, yellow, soft, asymptomatic papules with a central depression, located on the labia minora and inner aspects of the labia majora (Figures 7.1.9 and 7.1.10).

Definition: It is an appreciable enlargement of pilosebaceous units in nonectopic locations. Fordyce spots are heterotopic sebaceous glands that, similar to papillomatosis, are considered to be a physiologically asymptomatic condition.

Etiology: The pathogenesis of the proliferative abnormality leading to sebaceous hyperplasia is not fully understood. It is considered to be a hamartoma rather than a true neoplasm. Hormonal factors and chronic inflammation from HPV infection, previous surgery or ultraviolet exposure have been inconclusively considered among the possible cofactors of both conditions.

Epidemiology: True sebaceous hyperplasia is exceedingly rare, with only a few cases reported in the literature, whereas Fordyce spots are considered relatively common. Both conditions are more often observed in young adults.

Clinical course: They are benign conditions that persist indefinitely.

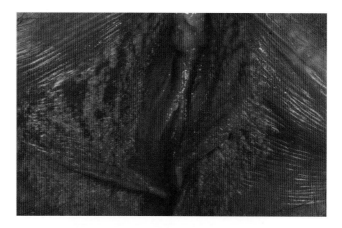

FIGURE 7.1.9   Multiple dome-shaped symmetrically distributed yellowish papules: Fordyce spots.

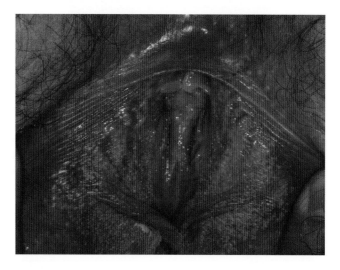

FIGURE 7.1.10   Fordyce spots.

Diagnosis: It is usually clinical, and histology is seldom required; dermoscopy shows a pattern characterized by aggregated white–yellowish globules.

Differential diagnosis: Molluscum contagiosum, nodular basal cell carcinoma, milia, and syringoma.

Therapy: These benign conditions do not require any treatment, unless cosmetic concerns raise the need for their surgical or laser ablation.

Bibliography

Al-Daraji WI, Wagner B, Ali RB. Sebaceous hyperplasia of the vulva: A clinicopathological case report with a review of the literature. *J Clin Pathol* 2007;60:835–7.

Niemann C. Differentiation of the sebaceous gland. *Dermatoendocrinol* 2009;1:64–7.

Ortiz-Rey JA, Martin-Jimenez A, Alvarez C, De La Fuente A. Sebaceous gland hyperplasia of the vulva. *Obstet Gynecol* 2002;99:919–21.

Zampeli VA, Makrantonaki E, Tzellos T, Zouboulis CC. New pharmaceutical concepts for sebaceous gland diseases: Implementing today's pre-clinical data into tomorrow's daily clinical practice. *Curr Pharm Biotechnol* 2012;13:1898–913.

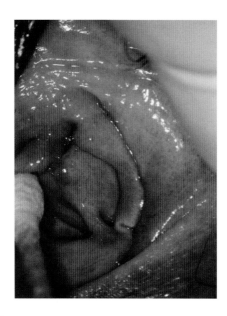

FIGURE 7.1.11   Urethral caruncle.

7.1.4 Urethral Caruncle

Clinical aspect: It most often appears as a pink or reddish asymptomatic exophytic papule at the urethral meatus (Figure 7.1.11); in rare cases, it may be purple or black secondary to thrombosis.

Definition: It is a benign, distal urethral lesion resulting from prolapse and ectropion of the urethral mucosa at the meatus.

Etiology: The cause is estrogen deficiency with consequent urogenital atrophy, which evolves into distal urethral prolapse.

Epidemiology: It is most commonly found in elderly postmenopausal women, but may rarely be observed in premenopausal or perimenopausal women.

Clinical course: Chronic irritation in the exposed mucosa contributes to the growth, hemorrhage, and eventual necrosis of the lesion, which may thus become painful, cause dysuria or, occasionally, bleed.

Diagnosis: A urethral caruncle is obvious on physical examination, and biopsy is unnecessary in the vast majority of cases. When the origin of the hematuria is uncertain, cystoscopy can be performed.

Differential diagnosis: The main differential diagnosis is with urethral prolapse.

Therapy: Warm baths, topical estrogens, and topical anti-inflammatory creams may be helpful. Surgical excision should be reserved to patients with larger symptomatic lesions in whom conservative therapy fails to elicit a response and to those with uncertain diagnosis.

Bibliography

Salim S, Taylor A, Carter C. Female paraphimosis? Management of a large female urethral caruncle, trialling manual reduction. *J Obstet Gynaecol* 2014;34:282–3.

Surabhi VR, Menias CO, George V, Siegel CL, Prasad SR. Magnetic resonance imaging of female urethral and periurethral disorders. *Radiol Clin North Am* 2013;51:941–53.

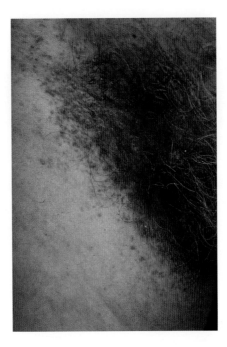

FIGURE 7.1.12   Multiple brownish and warty papules on the inguinal folds revealing Darier disease.

7.1.5 Darier Disease

Clinical aspect: Multiple, warty, crusted, yellow or brown papules involve the vulva and neighboring flexural areas (Figure 7.1.12), with the accumulation of foul-smelling keratotic debris, and typically develop also on the neck and upper thorax. Mucosal involvement may occur.

Definition: Inherited autosomal dominant disorder of keratinization occurring in the seborrheic areas of the body.

Etiology: It is due to a mutation of a gene located on band 2q23–24.1 causing a desmosomal disruption precipitated by heat, humidity, sweat, and friction.

Epidemiology: It is an uncommon disease (1/50,000) with equal frequency in males and females.

Clinical course: Onset is often at puberty. Extensive forms may cause considerable social handicap.

Diagnosis: The diagnosis is based on histological examination of the skin lesion biopsies revealing hyperkeratosis, focal dyskeratosis, and suprabasal acantholysis.

Differential diagnosis: Acanthosis nigricans, Hailey–Hailey disease, and bacterial infection (impetigo).

Therapy: The treatment is only symptomatic. Patients should avoid sun and heat. Emollients containing urea or lactic acid are of benefit for more limited lesions. Topical application of tretinoin or isotretinoin is effective against hyperkeratosis, but risk of irritation limits their use.

Bibliography

Adam AE. Ectopic Darier's disease of the cervix: An extraordinary cause of an abnormal smear. *Cytopathology* 1996;7:414–21.

Suárez-Peñaranda JM, Antúnez JR, Del Rio E, Vázquez VH, Novo Domínguez A. Vaginal involvement in a woman with Darier's disease: A case report. *Acta Cytol* 2005;49:530–2.

7.1.6 Angiokeratoma

Clinical aspect: Angiokeratomas appear as 1–5-mm, dome-shaped, grayish to purplish (caviar-like) and sometimes hyperkeratotic papules mainly located on the hair-bearing skin of the labia majora, and only rarely on the labia minora or clitoris (Figures 7.1.13 through 7.1.17). Patients are usually asymptomatic; vulvar itch, discomfort, burning, or pain are rarely reported.

Definition: It is a benign and localized proliferation and enlargement of dermal capillaries topped by a hyperkeratotic epithelium.

Etiology: In most cases, it appears spontaneously and without apparent cause. Underlying conditions that are sometimes proposed to play a pathogenetic role include venous hypertension, vascular fragility, and previous radiation therapy.

Epidemiology: Angiokeratomas are commonly observed on the external genitalia of adult subjects. In women, they are mostly reported at premenopausal age (<50 years).

Clinical course: Although they may increase in number and size over time, they are benign. Occasional bleeding secondary to traumas may occur. In rare cases, they can herald systemic disorders, such as Fabry's disease.

Diagnosis: The diagnosis is generally clinical, but may be supported by histopathology in selected cases to rule out other vascular tumors. At dermoscopy, a whitish veil and red or dark lacunae are common findings (Figure 7.1.18).

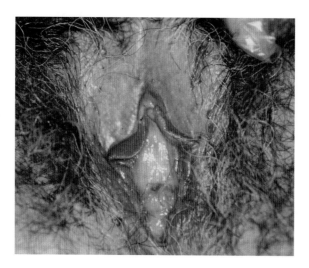

FIGURE 7.1.13   Reddish, dome-shaped papules: angiokeratomas.

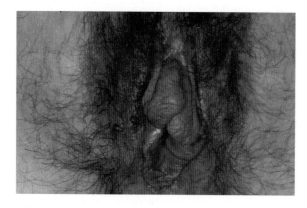

FIGURE 7.1.14   Purplish dome-shaped papules: multiple angiokeratomas.

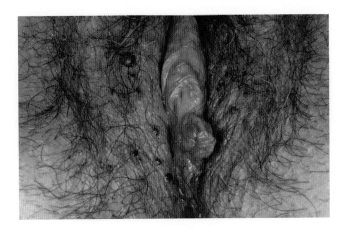

FIGURE 7.1.15   Multiple angiokeratomas.

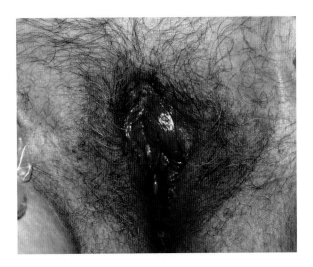

FIGURE 7.1.16   Multiple angiokeratomas.

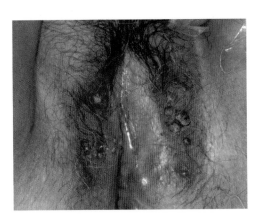

FIGURE 7.1.17   Multiple angiokeratomas.

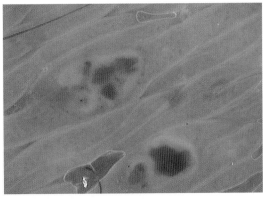

FIGURE 7.1.18   Dermoscopy of angiokeratomas: presence of dark lacunae and whitish veil.

Differential diagnosis: It includes Kaposi's sarcoma (KS), angiokeratoma of Mibelli, melanocytic nevi, melanoma, and anogenital warts. When occurring in teenagers or on extragenital sites, Fabry disease must be ruled out.

Therapy: No treatment is usually required. Bleeding or unesthetic lesions may be managed with laser therapy, electric coagulation, or cryotherapy, with liquid nitrogen.

Bibliography

Baruah J, Roy KK, Rahman SM, Kumar S, Pushparaj M, Mirdha AR. Angiokeratoma of vulva with coexisting human papilloma virus infection: A case report. *Arch Gynecol Obstet* 2008;278:165–7.

Buljan M. Multiple angiokeratomas of the vulva: Case report and literature review. *Acta Dermatovenerol Croat* 2010;18:271–5.

Micali G, Lacarrubba F. Augmented diagnostic capability using videodermatoscopy on selected infectious and non-infectious penile growths. *Int J Dermatol* 2011;50:1501–5.

Ozdemir M, Baysal I, Engin B, Ozdemir S. Treatment of angiokeratoma of Fordyce with long-pulse neodymium–yttrium aluminum garnet laser. *Dermatol Surg* 2009;35:92–7.

Pande SY, Kharkar VD, Mahajan S. Unilateral angiokeratoma of Fordyce. *Indian J Dermatol Venereol Leprol* 2004;70:377–9.

Smith BL, Chu P, Weinberg JM. Angiokeratomas of the vulva: Possible association with radiotherapy. *Skinmed* 2004;3:171–2.

Yigiter M, Arda IS, Tosun E, Celik M, Hiçsönmez A. Angiokeratoma of clitoris: A rare lesion in an adolescent girl. *Urology* 2007;71:604–6.

7.1.7 Seborrheic Keratosis

Clinical aspect: It may occur on the vulva as single or multiple roundish, sharply circumscribed, warty, yellowish–brown raised papules ranging in diameter from 2 to 10 mm (Figure 7.1.19). They may typically be covered by a greasy friable scale with a "stuck-on" appearance. No symptoms are reported, unless occasional mechanical traumas cause local inflammation or bleeding.

Definition: Commonly acquired, benign, pigmented, warty-surfaced epithelial proliferation that can appear anywhere on the body, except the palmoplantar areas. Synonyms for this condition are seborrheic wart and senile keratosis.

Etiology: It is unclear, but older age, family history, and sun exposure are considered to play a role.

Epidemiology: It is one of the most frequent skin tumors, but is uncommon on the vulva. It is mostly observed in Caucasians with no gender predilection, and its prevalence increases with advancing age.

Clinical course: They may increase in number and size or relapse after removal, but do not show any malignant potential.

Diagnosis: It is clinical. Dermoscopy shows milia-like cysts and comedo-like openings on a background varying from opaque light-brown to dark-brown or black (Figure 7.1.20). Histopathology may sometimes be required to rule out other hyperpigmented tumors.

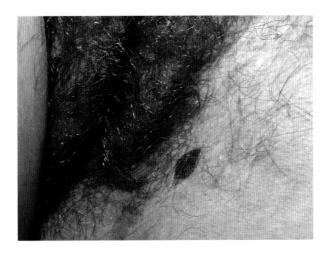

FIGURE 7.1.19 Sharply-circumscribed, brown and warty flat papule on the left inguinal fold: seborrheic keratosis.

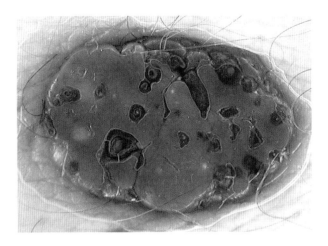

FIGURE 7.1.20 Dermoscopy of seborrheic keratosis: presence of milia-like cysts and comedo-like openings.

Differential diagnosis: Bowenoid papulosis, pigmented basal cell carcinoma, dermal melanocytic nevus, nodular melanoma, and verruciform xanthoma.

Therapy: Asymptomatic lesions need no treatment. If requested, removal may be performed by curettage, shaving, cryotherapy, electric cautery, or laser therapy.

Bibliography

De Giorgi V, Massi D, Salvini C. Pigmented seborrheic keratoses of the vulva clinically mimicking a malignant melanoma: A clinical, dermoscopic–pathologic case study. *Clin Exp Dermatol* 2005;30:17–9.

Keskin EA, Gorpelioglu C, Sarifakioglu E, Kafali H. Seborrheic keratoses: A distinctive diagnoses of pigmented vulvar lesions: A case report. *Cases J* 2010;3:56.

Reutter JC, Geisinger KR, Laudadio J. Vulvar seborrheic keratosis: Is there a relationship to human papillomavirus? *J Low Genit Tract Dis* 2014;18:190–4.

Shier RM, Rasty G. Vulvar seborrheic keratosis. *J Obstet Gynaecol Can* 2007;29:967–8.

Venkatesan A. Pigmented lesions of the vulva. *Dermatol Clin* 2010;28:795–805.

7.1.8 Bowenoid Papulosis

Clinical aspect: It can occur anywhere on the anogenital skin, but the most frequent localization in women is the vaginal labia. It presents with single or, more often, multiple isolated or grouped hyperpigmented, skin-colored or violaceous, flat, verrucous asymptomatic papules of a few millimeters to several centimeters in size (Figures 7.1.21 and 7.1.22).

Definition: It is a sexually transmitted precancerous skin condition of the genital area.

Etiology: It is a HPV-induced intraepithelial dysplasia (low-grade *in situ* carcinoma) mainly associated with HPV 16, but other types have also been found (HPV 18 and HPV 33).

Epidemiology: It is rare, and mostly affects young sexually active adults with a slight female predominance. It is more common in smokers and in HIV-positive individuals.

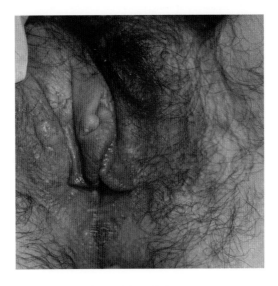

FIGURE 7.1.21   Multiple skin colored papules: bowenoid papulosis.

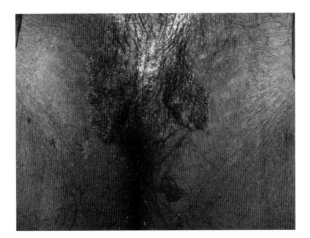

FIGURE 7.1.22   Multiple hyperpigmented, large and flat papules in a dark-skinned patient: bowenoid papulosis.

Clinical course: Though this condition is considered to be a low-grade *in situ* carcinoma, the prognosis is good in the majority of patients. Lesions may sometimes spontaneously regress. Evolution into an invasive squamous cell carcinoma more often occurs in immunosuppressed patients.

Diagnosis: Diagnosis is based on clinical and histological findings.

Differential diagnosis: Anogenital warts, seborrheic keratosis, Bowen's disease, pigmented basal cell carcinoma, and dermal melanocytic nevus.

Therapy: Treatment options include topical agents, such as 5-fluorouracil, imiquimod, podophyllin or cidofovir, and surgical modalities, such as excision, electrocautery, CO_2 laser, cryosurgery, and photodynamic therapy. Interferon and topical or systemic retinoids have also been tried with some success.

Bibliography

Campione E, Centonze C, Diluvio L, Orlandi A, Cipriani C, Di Stefani A, Piccione E, Chimenti S, Bianchi L. Bowenoid papulosis and invasive Bowen's disease: A multidisciplinary approach. *Acta Derm Venereol* 2013;93:228–9.

Shastry V, Betkerur J, Kushalappa. Bowenoid papulosis of the genitalia successfully treated with topical tazarotene. A report of two cases. *Indian J Dermatol* 2009;54:283–6.

Shim WH, Park HJ, Kim HS, Kim SH, Jung DS, Ko HC, Kim BS, Kim MB, Kwon KS. Bowenoid papulosis of the vulva and subsequent periungual Bowen's disease induced by the same mucosal HPVs. *Ann Dermatol* 2011;23:493–6.

7.2 Papules and/or Nodules

7.2.1 Pyogenic Granuloma

Clinical aspect: It clinically appears as a fast-growing and persistent, single or multiple, roundish, raised, sessile or pedunculated papule or nodule, usually ranging in diameter from a few millimeters to 2 cm, with a smooth or lobulated and bright red or purple surface (Figures 7.2.1 and 7.2.2). It is mostly painless, but may be slightly tender. This friable, polypoid lesion may sometimes show superficial ulcerations or cause bleeding after minor trauma.

Definition: It is a common and benign vascular proliferation of the skin and mucosa.

Etiology: It is still unclear, but is believed to be related to a reactive hyperproliferative vascular response to minor trauma and/or chronic low-grade local irritation, causing an excessive local production of angiogenic growth factors or cytokines that trigger endothelial proliferation and neoangiogenesis. Conditions reported in association with pyogenic granuloma are port-wine stain, insect bites, localized viral infections, psoriasis, eczema, burns, erythroderma, and cutaneous changes due to retinoid therapy.

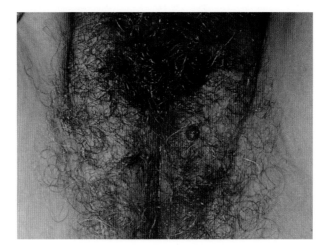

FIGURE 7.2.1 Single, purplish, raised and rapidly growing papule: pyogenic granuloma.

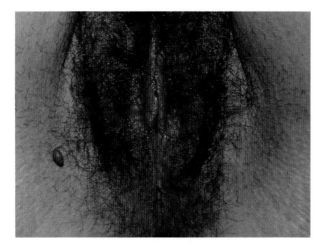

FIGURE 7.2.2 Pyogenic granuloma.

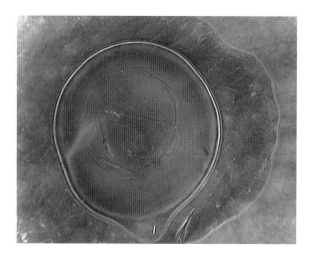

FIGURE 7.2.3 Dermoscopy of pyogenic granuloma: presence of reddish homogeneous area surrounded by a white collarette.

Epidemiology: Its incidence decreases with age, with a higher frequency reported in the first two decades of life and a slight female predilection.

Clinical course: Pyogenic granulomas of the vulva reported in the literature are all multiple and eruptive and grow rapidly over a few weeks. Untreated lesions may spontaneously regress, but only a minority completely clear, with residual atrophy within 6 months. Recurrence rates following treatment can be quite high (40%–50%).

Diagnosis: It is clinical. Videodermatoscopy showing red homogenous areas and intersecting whitish septa may be helpful (Figure 7.2.3). A biopsy to rule out other conditions is rarely necessary.

Differential diagnosis: This growth may closely resemble a nodular melanoma, but the short history, pedunculated growth, and epithelial collar are typical.

Therapy: Treatment options include curettage and cautery, cryotherapy, shave excision, excision with primary closure, and laser therapy.

Bibliography

Arikan DC, Kiran G, Sayar H, Kostu B, Coskun A, Kiran H. Vulvar pyogenic granuloma in a postmenopausal woman: Case report and review of the literature. *Case Rep Med* 2011;2011:201901.

Kaur T, Gupta S, Kumar B. Multiple pyogenic granuloma involving female genitalia: A rare entity? *Pediatr Dermatol* 2004;21:614–5.

Lee N, Isenstein A, Zedek D, Morrell DSA. A case of childhood subcutaneous pyogenic granuloma (lobular capillary hemangioma). *Clin Pediatr* 2012;51:88–90.

7.2.2 Dermal Melanocytic Nevus

Clinical aspect: Acquired dermal melanocytic nevi appear as usually small (<10 mm), circumscribed, raised, dome-shaped or flat, verrucous or polypoid, variably pigmented, soft or rubbery papules that, with time, may become more prominent and less pigmented because the clusters of nevus cells tend to settle deeper in the dermis (Figures 7.2.4 and 7.2.5). Congenital nevi may be larger (rarely giant) or show variable shapes with irregular well-defined edges (Figures 7.2.6 and 7.2.7).

Definition: Benign neoplasm or hamartoma characterized by the acquired or congenital accumulation of well-differentiated melanocytes in the superficial dermis.

Etiology: It remains unknown. It has been unequivocally proven that ultraviolet radiation is an inciting agent in the development of common acquired nevi on sun-exposed sites. However, nevi are known to develop on sun-protected sites, and genetic factors are considered to play an important role.

Epidemiology: Acquired melanocytic nevi are so common that some authorities believe they cannot be considered to be a defect or an abnormality. Most persons with light skin have at least a few. Dermal nevi are mostly observed by the third or fourth decade of life. In general, premenopausal women (aged 14–40 years) may present with this type of vulvar lesion. Congenital nevi are generally evident at birth.

Clinical course: It course is benign. Malignant transformation of dermal nevi is extremely rare. Giant congenital nevi (>20 cm) may be at risk for the development of malignant melanoma.

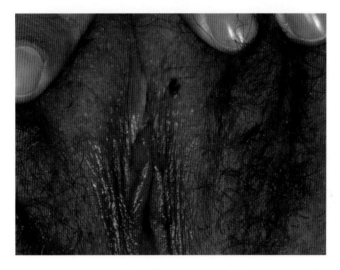

FIGURE 7.2.4 Flat, brown, slightly raised papules with regular edges: acquired dermal melanocytic nevus.

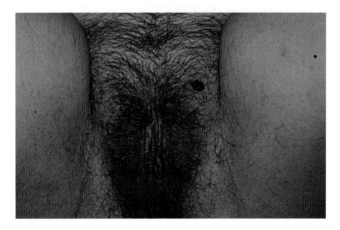

FIGURE 7.2.5 Acquired dermal melanocytic nevus.

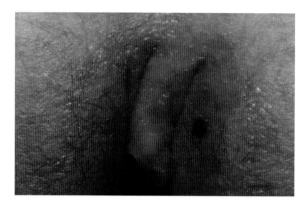

FIGURE 7.2.6   Flat, brown, slightly raised papule present since birth: congenital dermal melanocytic nevus.

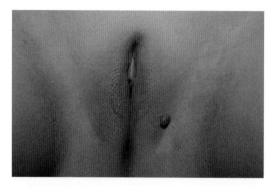

FIGURE 7.2.7   Congenital dermal melanocytic nevus mimicking acrochordon (see Section 9.1.3).

Diagnosis: It is primarily made by history and clinical presentation. Dermoscopy may be useful in differentiating benign nevi from other pigmented skin lesions (Figure 7.2.8). Histologic examination usually confirms the diagnosis in uncertain cases.

Differential diagnosis: Basal cell carcinoma, seborrheic keratosis, neurofibroma, trichoepithelioma, sebaceous hyperplasia, dermatofibroma, acrochordon, wart, nodular melanoma, clear cell acanthoma, and appendageal tumors.

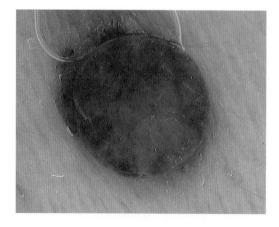

FIGURE 7.2.8   Dermoscopy of acquired dermal melanocytic nevus: presence of brown globules arranged in a cobblestone pattern.

Therapy: In most cases, no treatment is required. Suspicion that a nevus may be a melanoma, a change in the size, shape, or atypical pigmentation of the mole, chronic irritation or cosmetic concerns may prompt surgical excision.

Bibliography

El Shabrawi-Caelen L, Soyer HP, Schaeppi H, Cerroni L, Schirren CG, Rudolph C, Kerl H. Genital lentigines and melanocytic nevi with superimposed lichen sclerosus: A diagnostic challenge. *J Am Acad Dermatol* 2004;50:690–4.

Hengge UR, Meurer M. Pigmented lesions of the genital mucosa. *Hautarzt* 2005;56:540–9.

Ribé A. Melanocytic lesions of the genital area with attention given to atypical genital nevi. *J Cutan Pathol* 2008;35:24–7.

Schärer L. Melanocytic nevi at special anatomical sites. *Pathologie* 2007;28:430–6.

7.2.3 Endometriosis

Clinical aspect: In the vulva, it appears as an ill-defined, dark red, brown or blue–black cystic papule or nodule, usually located on the posterior fourchette, often showing cyclical variations in size according to menses (Figure 7.2.9). Cervical lesions may also occur (Figure 7.2.10). It is often painful, causing significant distress. Other reported symptoms include dysmenorrhea, heavy or irregular bleeding, pelvic or inguinal pain, dyspareunia, pain on micturition and/or urinary frequency, dyschezia (pain on defecation), diarrhea and constipation, bloating, nausea, and vomiting. A considerable percentage of cases are asymptomatic.

Definition: It consists of the presence of normal endometrial mucosa (glands and stroma) abnormally implanted in locations other than the uterine cavity.

Etiology: The exact cause is unclear. Suggested theories include the metaplastic conversion of celomic epithelium or the transport of endometrial cells through retrograde menstruation, but none have been entirely proven. This uncommon benign neoplasm may also be produced in the vulva by post-traumatic or postsurgical implantation of endometrial fragments.

Epidemiology: The most common sites of involvement are the ovaries, posterior cul-de-sac, and broad and uterosacral ligament. Vulvar lesions may occasionally occur.

Clinical course: Possible complications are infertility/subfertility and anatomic disruption of the involved organs (adhesions and ruptured cysts).

Diagnosis: Laparoscopy is considered to be the primary diagnostic modality for endometriosis. Histology can confirm the diagnosis.

Differential diagnosis: Appendicitis, gonorrhea and other chlamydial genitourinary infections, diverticulitis, ectopic pregnancy, ovarian cysts, and nodular melanoma.

Therapy: Treatment includes surgery and medical therapy with gonadotropin-releasing hormone analogs or oral contraceptive pills.

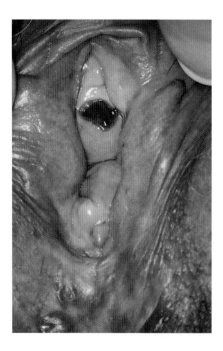

FIGURE 7.2.9 Indurated nodular plaques: Langerhans cell histiocytosis.

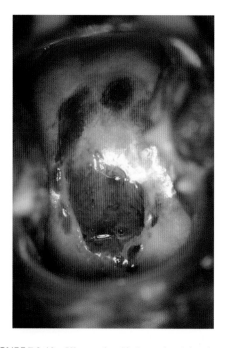

FIGURE 7.2.10 Ulcerated and indurated nodular plaques: Langerhans cell hisiocytosis.

Bibliography

Buda A, Ferrari L, Marra C, Passoni P, Perego P, Milani R. Vulvar endometriosis in surgical scar after excision of the Bartholin gland: Report of a case. *Arch Gynecol Obstet* 2008;277:255–6.

Gocmen A, Inaloz HS, Sari I. Endometriosis in the Bartholin gland. *Eur J Obstet Gynecol Reprod Biol* 2004;114:110–1.

Katz Z, Goldchmit R, Blickstein I. Post-traumatic vulvar endometriosis. *Eur J Pediatr Surg* 1996;6:241–2.

Nasu K, Okamoto M, Nishida M, Narahara H. Endometriosis of the perineum. *J Obstet Gynaecol Res* 2013;39:1095–7.

7.2.4 Langerhans Cell Histiocytosis

Clinical aspect: Female genital tract involvement is very rare and is usually seen as a part of multi-organ disease involving bone, skin, lymph nodes, brain, and lungs. The vulva is the most commonly involved genital site, although the disease has also been reported in the vagina, cervix, uterus, and ovaries. Clinically, most patients with vulvar involvement present with multiple ulcers or shallow erosions. However, vulvar lesions may take an extremely variable clinical presentation in the form of a pruritic rash, scaling, macular bruises, papules, nodules, or an area of induration (Figures 7.2.11 and 7.2.12).

Definition: It is a clonal neoplastic proliferation of bone marrow-derived Langerhans cells that may affect various tissues. Previously known as histiocytosis X, it includes a broad spectrum of clinical manifestations, namely eosinophilic granuloma, Hand–Schüller–Christian disease, and Letterer–Siwe disease.

Etiology: The underlying etiology is obscure. Immune system dysfunction related to cytokines, infectious agents, genetic factors, and neoplastic processes have all been considered.

Epidemiology: It is primarily regarded as a pediatric disease with a reported incidence of 1/200,000, although it may also occur in adults. Males are more commonly affected (male:female ratio = 3.7:1), but genital skin involvement is relatively more common in females. The mean age of presentation in women is 38 years. Focal lesions are generally diagnosed in older patients, particularly in postmenopausal women.

Clinical course: The clinical presentation and behavior of the disease varies greatly, ranging from mild to life-threatening. The prognosis is difficult to determine. There appears to be no correlation between the histology and the outcome of the genital lesions. Important factors for predicting disease recurrence and poor prognosis include young age (<5 years) at presentation and the disease involving three or more body systems and/or organ dysfunction. Spontaneous regression is possible in 10%–20% of patients.

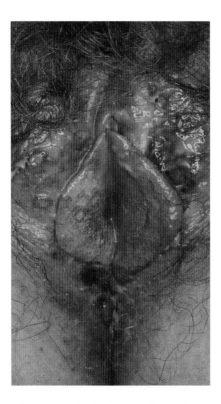

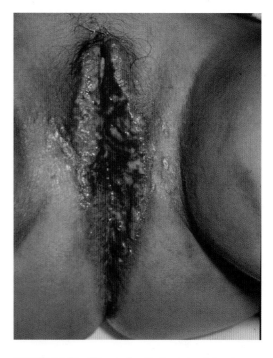

FIGURE 7.2.11   Indurated nodular plaques: Langerhans cell histiocytosis.

FIGURE 7.2.12   Ulcerated and indurated nodular plaques: Langerhans cell hisiocytosis.

Diagnosis: The gold standard for diagnosis is biopsy and histology with both hematoxylin–eosin and immunohistochemical staining for CD1a, S-100, or CD68.

Differential diagnosis: Due to its extremely varied clinical appearance, genital Langerhans cell histiocytosis may mimic various neoplastic and non-neoplastic conditions. Pruritic, erythematous lesions may resemble eczema or seborrheic dermatitis. Papular and ulcerated lesions may resemble chancroid, granuloma inguinale, lymphogranuloma venereum, syphilitic chancres, tuberculosis, herpes simplex, erythema multiforme, or Behçet's syndrome. It may be mistaken for cutaneous malignancies such as squamous cell carcinoma, melanoma, and sarcoma, particularly when presenting as a mass lesion. Diffusely indurated lesions clinically mimic extramammary Paget's disease.

Therapy: There is still no universally accepted treatment protocol available both for vulvar and systemic Langerhans cell histiocytosis. In the reported vulvar cases, vulvectomy, local excision, radiotherapy, chemotherapy, and topical and oral steroids were used as treatment options. Among them, complete surgical excision is the recommended treatment. Radiotherapy is also beneficial in some cases.

Bibliography

Ishigaki H, Hatta N, Yamada M, Orito H, Takehara K. Localized vulvar Langerhans cell histiocytosis. *Eur J Dermatol* 2004;14:412–4.

Kurt S, Canda MT, Kopuz A, Solakoglu Kahraman D, Tasyurt A. Diagnosis of primary Langerhans cell histiocytosis of the vulva in a postmenopausal woman. *Case Rep Obstet Gynecol* 2013;2013:962670.

Mottl H, Rob L, Stary J, Kodet R, Drahokoupilova E. Langerhans cell histiocytosis of vulva in an adolescent. *Int J Gynecol Cancer* 2007;17:520–4.

Pan Z, Sharma S, Sharma P. Primary Langerhans cell histiocytosis of the vulva: Report of a case and brief review of the literature. *Indian J Pathol Microbiol* 2009;52:65–8.

7.2.5 Metastases

Clinical aspect: The lesions most commonly present as grayish to red single papules and/or nodules, but multiple lesions may also be observed. They may be eroded or ulcerated (Figures 7.2.13 and 7.2.14) and are more often located around the labia minora and clitoris.

Definition: Metastasis or metastatic disease is the spread of a cancer from one organ or body part to another nonadjacent organ or body part. The most common tumors to metastasize to the vulva are squamous cell carcinomas of the cervix and adenocarcinomas of the endometrium.

Etiology: Implantation of metastatic tumor cells has been shown to be facilitated by the production of enzymes, such as proteinases and glycosidases, which are capable of degrading the various components of the extracellular matrix.

Epidemiology: The frequency of metastases changes according to tumor type. Vulvar metastases are mostly recorded in advanced age.

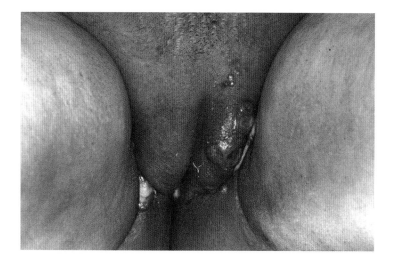

FIGURE 7.2.13   Multiple nodules and papules on a background of radiation dermatitis: vulvar metastases from rectal adenocarcinoma.

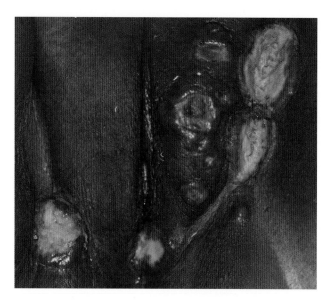

FIGURE 7.2.14   A detail of the same patient showing prominent ulceration.

Clinical course: Prognosis is poor. Genital involvement is usually associated with disseminated disease, and the average survival after the detection of cutaneous metastasis is usually only 3 months.

Diagnosis: It is usually made by histological examination. At times, cell differentiation and architectural structure allow for the identification of the primary tumor site; however, the cells are often anaplastic.

Differential diagnosis: Keloid, lymphoma, sarcoidosis, and primary invasive carcinomas.

Therapy: Treatment depends on the primary tumor. With solitary or few lesions, surgical excision may be performed. In terminal patients, only palliative or supportive therapy is indicated.

Bibliography

Abdullah A, Seagle BL, Bautista E, Hansra BS, Samuelson R, Shahabi S. Vulvar metastasis of an early-stage well-differentiated endometrial cancer after minimally invasive surgery. *J Minim Invasive Gynecol* 2014;21:708–11.

Androulaki A, Papathomas TG, Alexandrou P, Lazaris AC. Metastatic low-grade endometrial stromal sarcoma of clitoris: Report of a case. *Int J Gynecol Cancer* 2007;17:290–3.

Hoyt BS, Cohen PR. Reply to: A rare case of vulvar skin metastasis of rectal cancer after operation. *Int J Dermatol* 2014;53:e339–40.

7.3 Inflammatory Papules and/or Plaques

7.3.1 Lichen Planus

Clinical aspect: Most cases occur in the setting of extensive cutaneous involvement as typical multiple, isolated or confluent, flat, polyhedral, lilaceous and shiny papules or plaques on the genital skin of the labia and mons pubis (Figures 7.3.1 through 7.3.3). The concomitant presence of whitish reticular mucosal streaks (Wickham's striae) is almost a rule (Figures 7.3.4 through 7.3.6). An erosive and destructive form (vulvovaginal–gingival syndrome) (Figure 7.3.7), resulting in atrophy or scarring, has also been described (see also Section 7.3.9). Less commonly, a rare hypertrophic form, characterized by raised whitish warty plaques with pronounced hyperkeratosis and frequent extensive scarring of the periclitoral area, may be observed. Itching and irritation, which is particularly severe in the hypertrophic variant, are frequently reported. A burning sensation and dyspareunia are also common. Erosive forms may be very painful.

Definition: It is a chronic cutaneous and/or mucosal inflammatory disorder related to immunological dysregulation that may affect the oral cavity and genitalia.

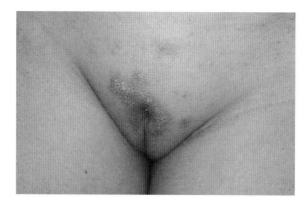

FIGURE 7.3.1   Lilac cutaneous pruritic papules with superficial whitish reticular streaks: lichen planus.

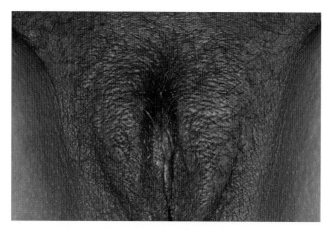

FIGURE 7.3.2   Lichen planus: extensive vulvar involvement.

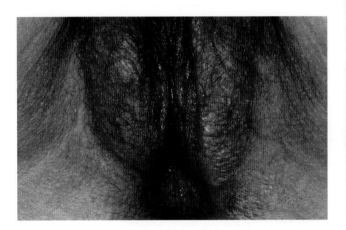

FIGURE 7.3.3 Vulvar lichen planus with prominent cutaneous thickening.

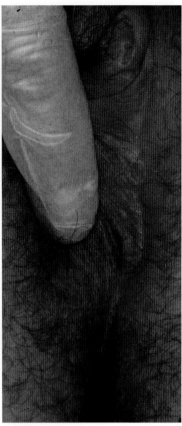

FIGURE 7.3.4 Whitish circinated streaks: lichen planus.

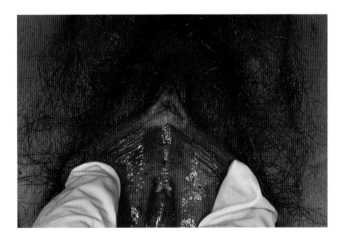

FIGURE 7.3.5 Whitish adherent mucosal patches: lichen planus.

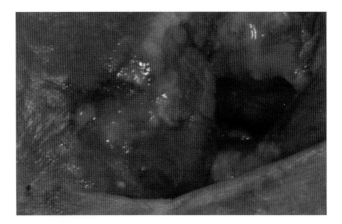

FIGURE 7.3.6   Lichen planus: mucosal involvement.

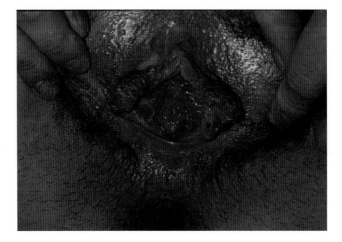

FIGURE 7.3.7   Shallow erosions with whitish streaks: erosive lichen planus (see also Section 7.7.1).

Etiology: It is likely to be a T cell-mediated immune response to an unknown antigen resulting in an epidermotropic lymphocytic infiltrate. It may be found with other diseases of altered immunity, such as alopecia areata, vitiligo, thyroid disease, ulcerative colitis, dermatomyositis, morphea, lichen sclerosus, myasthenia gravis, and primary biliary cirrhosis. An association is noted between lichen planus and hepatitis C virus infection.

Epidemiology: It is reported in approximately 1% of all new patients seen at health care clinics. No significant geographical variations in frequency and no racial predispositions have been noted. Although it can occur at any age, more than two-thirds of patients are aged 30–60 years. Vulvar involvement is not rare and is reported in more than 50% of women with generalized disease.

Clinical course: The classic papular variant usually clears within 6 (>50%) to 18 months (85%) with no atrophy or scarring. Vulvar scarring and urethral stenosis may be a complication of the erosive and hypertrophic variants, which are usually long-standing and poorly responsive to treatment, showing an indolent, chronic, and often disabling course.

Diagnosis: Diagnosis is clinical in most cases, and may be supported by the finding of typical lesions in the oral cavity or other skin areas. Dermoscopy may show pearly whitish structures that are comb-like or arboriform projections corresponding to the Wickham striae (Figure 7.3.8). In case of unspecific features, skin biopsy is indicated.

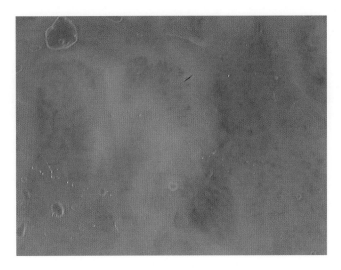

FIGURE 7.3.8 Dermoscopy of lichen planus: presence of whitish areas surrounded by radial capillaries.

Differential diagnosis: Lichen sclerosus, lichen simplex chronicus, psoriasis, dermatophytosis, lupus erythematosus, and, for erosive lichen planus, autoimmune blistering disorders (cicatricial or bullous pemphigoid, and pemphigus).

Therapy: Mild cases can be managed with potent topical steroids; topical calcineurin inhibitors may be used as an alternative, second-line option. More severe cases may require a more intensive treatment with systemic corticosteroids or oral cyclosporine. Other reportedly effective treatments include topical or oral retinoids, metronidazole, sulfasalazine, mycophenolate mofetil, and phototherapy (narrowband or broadband ultraviolet B or psoralen combined with ultraviolet A treatment).

Bibliography

Belfiore P, Di Fede O, Cabibi D, Campisi G, Amarù GS, De Cantis S, Maresi E. Prevalence of vulval lichen planus in a cohort of women with oral lichen planus: An interdisciplinary study. *Br J Dermatol* 2006;155:994–8.

Di Fede O, Belfiore P, Cabibi D, De Cantis S, Maresi E, Kerr AR, Campisi G. Unexpectedly high frequency of genital involvement in women with clinical and histological features of oral lichen planus. *Acta Derm Venereol* 2006;86:433–8.

Lewis FM. Vulval lichen planus. *Br J Dermatol* 1998;138:569–75.

Lewis FM, Shah M, Harrington CI. Vulval involvement in lichen planus: A study of 37 women. *Br J Dermatol* 1996;135:89–91.

Thorstensen KA, Birenbaum DL. Recognition and management of vulvar dermatologic conditions: Lichen sclerosus, lichen planus, and lichen simplex chronicus. *J Midwifery Women's Health* 2012;57:260–75.

Vázquez-López F. Lichen ruber planus. In: Micali G, Lacarrubba F (eds). *Dermatoscopy in Clinical Practice: Beyond Pigmented Lesions*. Informa Healthcare Ltd, London (UK), 2010.

7.4 Vascular Papules and/or Plaques

7.4.1 Hemangioma

Clinical aspect: It is usually observed at birth as macules of erythema of variable size that rapidly progress in the following months to well-circumscribed, raised, red and soft papules or plaques. Most lesions are observed on the labia majora (Figures 7.4.1 through 7.4.5), but other areas, including the labia minora, the perineum, and the perianal region, may be affected (Figure 7.4.6).

Definition: It is a benign congenital vascular proliferation of the endothelial cells that line the blood vessels, characterized by an increased number of normal or abnormal vessels filled with blood.

Etiology: Its cause is currently unknown; however, several studies point to a role of estrogen signaling in the induction of vascular proliferation.

Epidemiology: Hemangiomas are the most common tumors of infancy. Although their precise incidence is unknown, they are classically said to occur in up to 10% of Caucasian infants.

Clinical course: Over time, these lesions almost entirely regress, leaving a usually barely appreciable fibrotic scar. Possible complications include ulceration, bleeding, urethral obstruction and, in case of large hemangiomas, consumptive coagulopathy (Kasabach–Merritt syndrome).

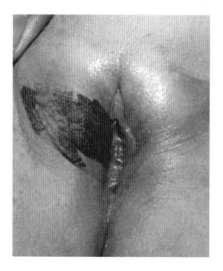

FIGURE 7.4.1   Flat, smooth and soft reddish plaque with sharp edges: hemangioma.

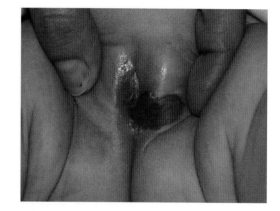

FIGURE 7.4.2   Hemangioma.

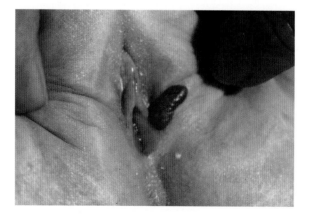

FIGURE 7.4.3   Hemangioma.

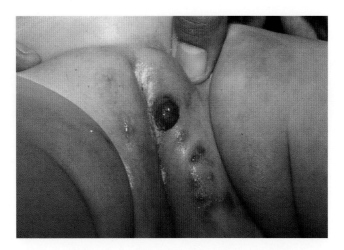

FIGURE 7.4.4 Raised, reddish, dome-shaped progressively enlarging lesion: hemangioma.

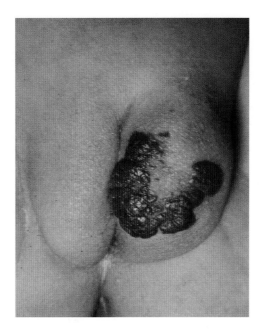

FIGURE 7.4.5 Hemangioma with associated deep involvement.

Diagnosis: It is usually made on clinical grounds.

Differential diagnosis: Angiokeratoma, pyogenic granuloma, bacillary angiomatosis, hemangiopericytoma, angiosarcoma, and Kaposi's sarcoma (KS).

Therapy: An attending approach is recommended, since spontaneous resolution is almost a rule. Treatment is indicated in patients who are at risk of urinary obstruction or in case of extensive ulceration and bleeding. Medical treatments include intralesional or systemic corticosteroids, interferon and, more recently, beta-blockers. Surgical treatment is best performed by neodymium–yttrium aluminum garnet laser therapy.

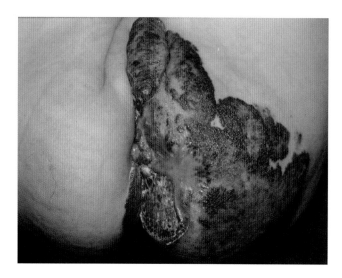

FIGURE 7.4.6   Extensive and ulcerated hemangioma with vulvoperineal and gluteal involvement.

Bibliography

Bava GL, Dalmonte P, Oddone M, Rossi U. Life-threatening hemorrhage from a vulvar hemangioma. *J Pediatr Surg* 2002;37:E6.

Bruni V, Pontello V, Dei M, Alessandrini M, Li Marzi V, Nicita G. Hemangioma of the clitoris presenting as clitoromegaly: A case report. *J Pediatr Adolesc Gynecol* 2009;22:e137–8.

Mouhari-Toure A, Azoumah KD, Tchamdja K, Saka B, Kombaté K, Tchangaï-Walla K, Pitche P. Rapid regression of infantile haemangioma with 2% propranolol ointment. *Ann Dermatol Venereol* 2013;140:462–4.

7.4.2 Kaposi's Sarcoma

Clinical aspect: KS often involves the genitalia as part of a disseminated cutaneous disease. Lesions may have a macular, papular, nodular, or plaque-like appearance (Figures 7.4.7 and 7.4.8). They may range in size from a few millimeters to several centimeters and may assume a pink, red, brown, or violaceous color, which may be difficult to distinguish in dark-skinned individuals. Nearly all lesions are palpable and nonpruritic. Ulceration may be present. Vulvar lesions may occasionally cause interference with urinary flow.

Definition: It is a spindle-cell tumor that is thought to be derived from endothelial cell lineage. It can be primarily categorized into four types: classic (sporadic Mediterranean), epidemic (AIDS-related), iatrogenic (in transplanted immunosuppressed patients), and endemic (African).

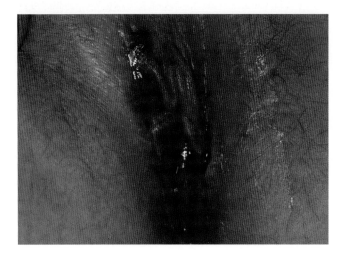

FIGURE 7.4.7   Kaposi's sarcoma.

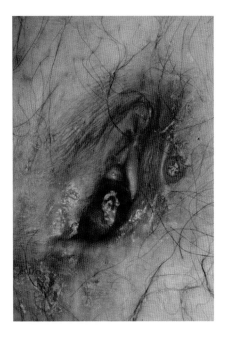

FIGURE 7.4.8   Kaposi's sarcoma.

Etiology: Herpes virus type 8 (KSHV or HHV8) is now recognized as the causative agent and is present in more than 90% of all variants of KS. This viral infection may be transmitted, usually early in life, by saliva, or later on by sexual contact. Factors that are thought to stimulate the secretion of autocrine and paracrine vascular endothelial growth factors leading to KS development include an abnormal cytokine milieu that may be associated with cellular and humoral immunity defects or HIV infection.

Epidemiology: AIDS-related KS is the most common presentation of vulvar KS. Before the AIDS epidemic, vulvar KS was very rare.

Clinical course: This condition carries a variable clinical course ranging from minimal mucocutaneous disease to a more rapidly disseminated disease with extensive organ involvement. AIDS-related KS, unlike the classic variant, tends to have an aggressive clinical course.

Diagnosis: Typical clinical features may suggest the diagnosis, which is usually confirmed by histological examination.

Differential diagnosis: Hemangioma, angiokeratoma, pyogenic granuloma, bacillary angiomatosis, hemangiopericytoma, and angiosarcoma.

Therapy: Treatment depends on the clinical type and on the disease staging. Optimal control of HIV infection using highly active antiretroviral therapy is an integral part of successful AIDS-related KS therapy. The following local therapies can be used for the palliation of locally advanced symptomatic disease or in individuals who have cosmetically unacceptable lesions: radiation therapy, cryotherapy, neodymium–yttrium aluminum garnet laser therapy, surgical excision, intralesional vinca alkaloid therapy, topical retinoids, and interferon-alfa.

Bibliography

D'Antuono A, Zauli S, Bellavista S, Banzola N, Rech G, Balestri R, Patrizi A. AIDS-related Kaposi's sarcoma involving the genital and inguinal regions. *Int J Dermatol* 2013;52:1435–7.

Laartz BW, Cooper C, Degryse A, Sinnott JT. Wolf in sheep's clothing: Advanced Kaposi sarcoma mimicking vulvar abscess. *South Med J* 2005;98:475–7.

Riggs RM, McCarthy J. Vulvar Kaposi's sarcoma in a woman with AIDS: A case report. *J Reprod Med* 2005;50:730–2.

Schwartz RA, Micali G, Nasca MR, Scuderi L. Kaposi's sarcoma: A continuing conundrum. *J Am Acad Dermatol* 2008;59:179–206.

7.5 Vascular Papules and/or Plaques plus Vesicles

7.5.1 Lymphangioma

Clinical aspect: Primary vulvar involvement is rarely observed on the labia minora or majora as raised, compressible, doughy papules or plaques that are typically heralded (lymphangioma circumscriptum) by a persistent superficial noninflammatory blistering, with multiple clustered, small, thin-walled and translucent pseudovesicles filled with clear fluid ("frog-spawn") (Figures 7.5.1 and 7.5.2). No symptoms have been reported.

Definition: Lymphangiomas are uncommon, benign, congenital, lymphatic malformations (hamartomas) of the lymphatic system.

Etiology: This congenital abnormality of the lymphatic system is probably due to sequestration of lymphatic tissue during embryogenesis as a result of a failure to establish a connection with the normal network of drainage vessels. In some instances, secondary causes, such as damage and obstruction of the deep lymphatic collecting channels with consequent lymph stasis and dilation of the upper dermal

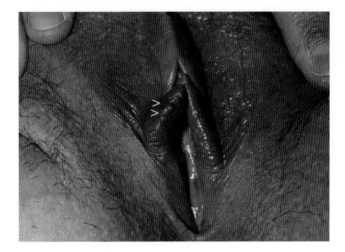

FIGURE 7.5.1   Pseudovesicles (arrows) in lymphangioma circumscriptum.

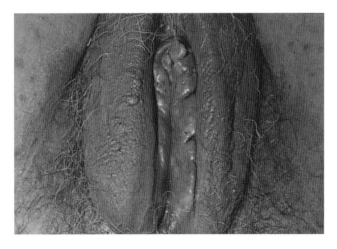

FIGURE 7.5.2   Pseudovesicles (arrows) with lymphedema: lymphangioma circumscriptum.

lymphatics (from traumas, inflammatory disorders, surgery, or radiation therapy), have been claimed to play a role.

Epidemiology: It is rare and accounts for approximately 5% of all vascular tumors in children. It is usually present at birth or develops early in infancy, but secondary forms more often occur in adulthood.

Clinical course: In most cases, this is a benign and often negligible condition. Follow-up of patients with lymphoedema is recommended because transformation to lymphangiosarcoma may rarely occur.

Diagnosis: If the clinical diagnosis is difficult, histological identification may be performed. Ultrasonography may be helpful to rule out deep extension.

Differential diagnosis: Anogenital warts, molluscum contagiosum, and cysts.

Therapy: If needed, surgical removal or CO_2 laser vaporization may be performed with acceptable cosmetic results. Incomplete excision may result in recurrence.

Bibliography

Ikeda M, Muramatsu T, Shida M, Hirasawa T, Ishimoto H, Izumi S, Mikami M. Surgical management of vulvar lymphangioma circumscriptum: Two case reports. *Tokai J Exp Clin Med* 2011;36:17–20.

Kokcu A, Yildiz L, Bildircin D, Kandemir B. Vulvar lymphangioma circumscriptum presenting periodic symptoms. *BMJ Case Rep* 2010; doi: 10.1136/bcr.06.2010.3056.

Stewart CJ, Chan T, Platten M. Acquired lymphangiectasia ('lymphangioma circumscriptum') of the vulva: A report of eight cases. *Pathology* 2009;41:448–53.

Tulasi NR, John A, Chauhan I. Lymphangioma circumscriptum. *Int J Gynecol Cancer* 2004;14:564–6.

Uçmak D, Aytekin S, Sula B, Akkurt ZM, Türkçü G, Ağaçayak E. Acquired vulvar lymphangioma circumscriptum. *Case Rep Dermatol Med* 2013;2013:967890.

Watanabe T, Matsubara S, Yamaguchi T, Yamanaka Y. Cavernous lymphangiomas involving bilateral labia minora. *Obstet Gynecol* 2010;116:510–2.

7.6 Proliferative Papules and/or Plaques

7.6.1 Epidermal Nevus/Inflammatory Linear Verrucous Epidermal Nevus (ILVEN)

Clinical aspect: Most commonly, it involves an extremity or, at times, other areas. The vulva may occasionally be affected (Figures 7.6.1 and 7.6.2). It is characterized by intensely erythematous, pruritic, and inflammatory papules or plaques that occur as linear bands along the lines of Blaschko.

Definition: It is a benign cutaneous hamartoma.

Etiology: It is unknown. It is regarded as a localized dyskeratotic disease reflecting genetic mosaicism.

Epidemiology: A female predominance is reported for ILVEN (female:male ratio = 4:1).

Clinical course: It is usually uneventful. If untreated, these lesions persist indefinitely.

Diagnosis: Diagnosis is clinical, but may be confirmed by histology.

Differential diagnosis: Darier disease, lichen simplex chronicus, and lichen planus.

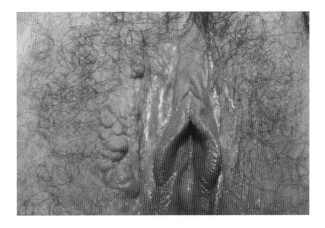

FIGURE 7.6.1 Multiple raised proliferative papules present since birth: epidermal nevus.

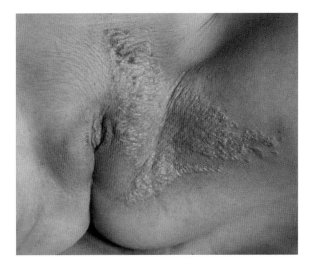

FIGURE 7.6.2 ILVEN.

Therapy: Treatment is not recommended unless the lesion is very bothersome. In such cases, CO_2 laser therapy can be attempted.

Bibliography

Le K, Wong LC, Fischer G. Vulval and perianal inflammatory linear verrucous epidermal naevus. *Australas J Dermatol* 2009;50:115–7.

Molin L, Särhammar G. Perivulvar inflammatory linear verrucous epidermal nevus (ILVEN) treated with CO_2 laser. *J Cutan Laser Ther* 1999;1:53–6.

Nag F, Ghosh A, Surana TV, Biswas S, Gangopadhyay A, Chatterjee G. Inflammatory linear verrucous epidermal nevus in perineum and vulva: A report of two rare cases. *Indian J Dermatol* 2013;58:158.

7.6.2 Secondary Syphilis

Clinical aspect: It is characterized by multiple signs and symptoms, which most commonly involve the skin, mucous membranes, and lymph nodes. On the skin, subentrant maculopapular and papulosquamous symmetrical and nonitchy rashes develop over the trunk, the extremities, and typically on the palms and soles. Wart-like, rounded, flattened, grayish, soft, oozing papules and vegetating plaques, known as condylomata lata, arise in the vulvar and perianal areas and may also affect the mouth (Figures 7.6.3 and 7.6.4). Generalized lymphoadenopathy, malaise, headache, sore throat, arthralgia, and hair loss usually appear.

Definition: Syphilis is a sexually transmitted disease that predominantly affects the genital area and is characterized by different clinical stages. Secondary syphilis is the second disease stage, following unaware primary syphilis, which occurs after an asymptomatic latent period of approximately 10 weeks.

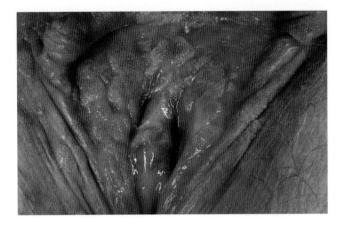

FIGURE 7.6.3 Condylomata lata: secondary syphilis.

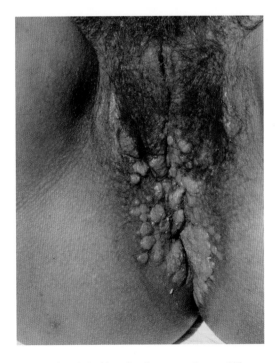

FIGURE 7.6.4 Multiple raised plaques in a dark-skinned patient: secondary syphilis.

Etiology: It reflects the generalization of the sexually transmitted infection caused by *Treponema pallidum.*

Epidemiology: Syphilis is diffused worldwide, with the highest rates in many developing countries (South and South-East Asia, sub-Saharan Africa, Latin America, and Eastern Europe). In recent years, its incidence has been rising in the Western world, especially in metropolitan areas and among homosexual men. Secondary syphilis develops in approximately a third of untreated individuals with primary syphilis, but many women (40%–85%) do not report having had the classic chancre previously.

Clinical course: The lesions develop slowly and can persist for weeks or months with few symptoms. Recurrence is reported in approximately 25% of patients. This secondary period lasts for 2–3 years before entering the late, tertiary stage.

Diagnosis: A positive dark-field examination of a swab obtained from the mucous membrane lesions is diagnostic. VDRL and RPR serology shows high titers. In early secondary syphilis, tests may be falsely negative, so FTA-ABS tests are required.

Differential diagnosis: Anogenital warts.

Therapy: First-line treatment is penicillin injection, used at the same dosages as for primary syphilis if the disease duration is less than 1 year, or longer in diseases with durations of more than 1 year. Concurrent systemic steroid administration is recommended to prevent Jarisch–Herxheimer reactions. In case of penicillin allergy, erythromycin or doxycycline may be used. VDRL and TPHA titration are useful for post-treatment follow-up.

Bibliography

Boudhir H, Ellouadghiri A, Mael-Ainin M, Hassam B. Secondary syphilis revealed by palmar keratoderma and vegetating vulvar lesions. *Ann Dermatol Venereol* 2012;139:864–5.

Fiumara NJ. Unusual location of condyloma lata. A case report. *Br J Vener Dis* 1977;53:391–3.

Mullooly C, Higgins SP. Secondary syphilis: The classical triad of skin rash, mucosal ulceration and lymphadenopathy. *Int J STD AIDS* 2010;21:537–45.

7.6.3 Condyloma (Anogenital Warts)

Clinical aspect: They are often multiple and appear as raised, pedunculated or sessile, skin-colored, pink or brown, warty, soft papules of variable sizes, which may become confluent as outgrowing cauliflower-like plaques (Figures 7.6.5 through 7.6.12). They frequently occur on the introitus, vagina, labia, perineum, or pubic skin.

Definition: Condylomas represent a common sexually transmissible disorder affecting the genital area due to a HPV infection.

Etiology: Genital involvement is linked to mucosal HPV types, which most commonly include the low-risk nononcogenic HPV 6 and 11 types. Less common causative agents are high-risk oncogenic types, such as HPV 16 and 18.

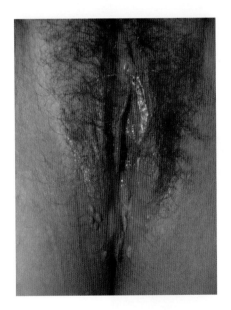

FIGURE 7.6.5 Multiple clustered skin-colored and soft papules: anogenital warts.

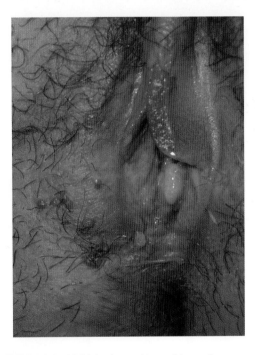

FIGURE 7.6.6 Multiple clustered brownish papules: anogenital warts.

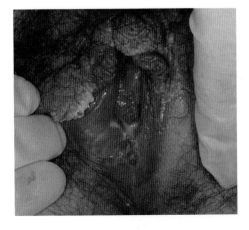

FIGURE 7.6.7 Cauliflower-like plaques: anogenital warts.

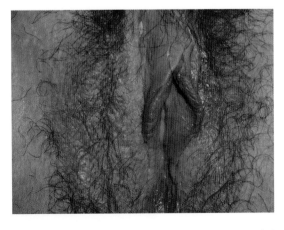

FIGURE 7.6.8 Flat whitish verrucous plaque: anogenital warts.

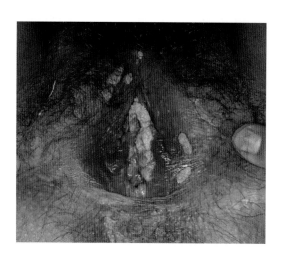

FIGURE 7.6.9   Anogenital warts: multiple lesions.

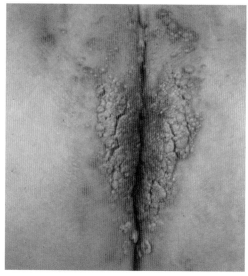

FIGURE 7.6.10   Papules and verrucous plaques: anogenital warts.

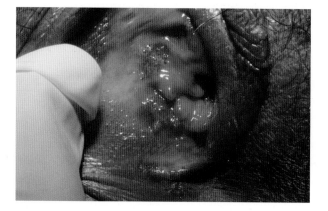

FIGURE 7.6.11   Anogenital warts: mucosal lesions.

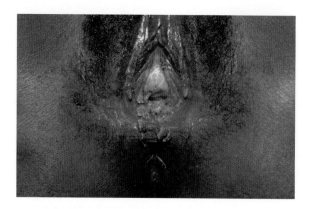

FIGURE 7.6.12   Anogenital warts in a dark-skinned patient.

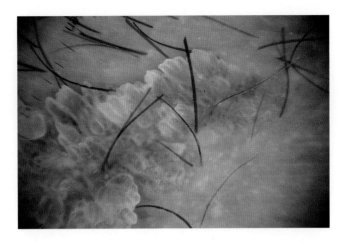

FIGURE 7.6.13 Dermoscopy of anogenital warts: presence of irregular papillomatous projections with elongated vessels.

Epidemiology: Anogenital warts are reported worldwide at similar rates in both sexes, with a variable annual prevalence in females of as high as 120/100,000. Their incidence peaks before 24 years of age.

Clinical course: Spontaneous healing may occur, but progressive enlarging in untreated cases is almost the rule. In addition, concurrent cervical infection is likely in women with vulvar lesions. When high-risk oncogenic HPVs are the causative agents, a vulvar squamous cell carcinoma may develop later on.

Diagnosis: Careful clinical observation and past medical history are usually diagnostic. Identification of a mosaic (whitish network circumscribing areas centered by dilated glomerular vessels) or finger-like (whitish irregular projections including dilated and elongated vessels) pattern on dermoscopy may be helpful (Figure 7.6.13), whereas the application of acetic acid solution is no longer considered reliable for identifying subclinical infection, but may be useful for addressing the biopsy in some of those rare cases in which histological confirmation is required. HPV DNA testing is available and may be performed in selected cases.

Differential diagnosis: Depending on their size and clinical features, anogenital warts may mimic papillomatosis, Fordyce spots, acrochordons, molluscum contagiosum, secondary syphilis (condylomata lata), bowenoid papulosis, Buschke–Loewenstein tumor (verrucous carcinoma), or invasive carcinomas.

Therapy: Medical treatment may be performed with immune response modifiers (imiquimod 5% cream) or cytotoxic agents (podophyllotoxin 0.15% cream or trichloroacetic acid). Physical destruction methods include electrosurgery, cryosurgery, laser treatment, and surgical excision.

Bibliography

Ljubojevic S, Skerlev M. HPV-associated diseases. *Clin Dermatol* 2014;32:227–34.

Lynde C, Vender R, Bourcier M, Bhatia N. Clinical features of external genital warts. *J Cutan Med Surg* 2013;2:S55–60.

Nelson EL, Stockdale CK. Vulvar and vaginal HPV disease. *Obstet Gynecol Clin North Am* 2013;40:359–76.

7.6.4 Verrucous Carcinoma

Clinical aspect: It appears as an exophytic, cauliflower-like vegetant papule or plaque located in the external genitalia (Figures 7.6.14 and 7.6.15). It is usually itchy and sometimes painful.

Definition: It is a low-grade variant of squamous cell carcinoma primarily affecting the genitals in both sexes.

Etiology: The etiology is unclear, but this tumor has often been associated with the presence of low-risk HPV 6 and 11 in the neoplastic tissue.

Epidemiology: It is a rare tumor, overall constituting less than 1% of vulvar cancers. It occurs more frequently in women with a primary squamous epithelial cancer in another site of the female genital tract, especially the cervix, which shares with the vulva a common embryologic origin from the cloaco-genic membrane.

Clinical course: This well-differentiated neoplasm is locally invasive and may frequently extend into deep adjacent structures, but, as a rule, it does not cause distant metastases. Therefore, its prognosis is relatively good if wide local excision is performed.

Diagnosis: It may be difficult to diagnose from insufficiently large biopsies, resulting in misdiagnosis and inappropriate treatment.

Differential diagnosis: Anogenital warts, squamous cell carcinoma, hypertrophic lichen planus, and lichen simplex chronicus.

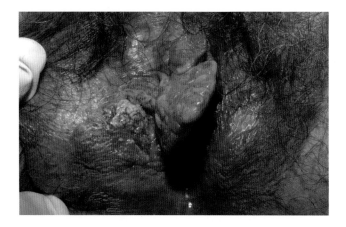

FIGURE 7.6.14   Vegetant plaque: verrucous carcinoma.

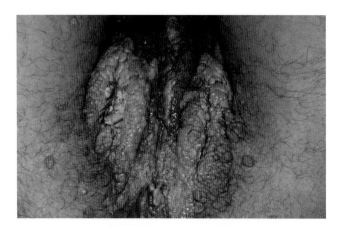

FIGURE 7.6.15   Cauliflower-like and cerebriform massive vegetation: verrucous carcinoma.

Therapy: Surgery is considered the most effective treatment, but it can be associated with local recurrences, especially when the tumor has been inadequately resected. Radiation therapy is poorly effective and may cause anaplastic transformation into a squamous cell carcinoma.

Bibliography

Boutas I, Sofoudis C, Kalampokas E, Anastasopoulos C, Kalampokas T, Salakos N. Verrucous carcinoma of the vulva: A case report. *Case Rep Obstet Gynecol* 2013;2013:932712.

Carter JS, Downs LS Jr. Vulvar and vaginal cancer. *Obstet Gynecol Clin North Am* 2012;39:213–31.

Isaacs JH. Verrucous carcinoma of the female genital tract. *Gynecol Oncol* 1976;4:259–69.

Lorente AI, Morillo M, de Zulueta T, Gonzalez J, Conejo-Mir J. Verrucous squamous cell carcinoma of vulva simulating multiple epidermal inclusion cysts. *Indian J Dermatol* 2013;58:318–9.

7.7 Ulcerative Papules and/or Plaques

7.7.1 Erosive Lichen Planus

Clinical aspect: Eroded papules or plaques often showing a white "lacy" edge are seen in the vulvo-vaginal area at the fourchette and extend to the anterior vestibule (Figures 7.7.1 through 7.7.3). Frequent symptoms are soreness, severe burning, and pain, often causing dysuria and dyspareunia. Patients with vaginal involvement may complain of a vaginal discharge that may be blood stained.

Definition: It is a chronic, painful condition affecting mucosal surfaces, mainly the mouth (oral lichen planus) and the genitals (vulval or penile lichen planus). This clinical form is often variably defined as ulcerative lichen planus, desquamative inflammatory vaginitis, or (when concomitant oral involvement is present) vulvovaginal–gingival syndrome.

Etiology: Evidence points to lichen planus being a T cell-mediated autoimmune inflammatory disease, but the antigen triggering the T lymphocyte response has not been identified. Basal keratinocyte degeneration is thought to be due to CD8⁺ T lymphocytes. Associations with other autoimmune diseases (alopecia areata, vitiligo, and thyroid disease) and hepatitis C infection have been reported.

Epidemiology: The prevalence of erosive lichen planus in the general population is unknown, but this is considered the most common clinical variant affecting the genitalia.

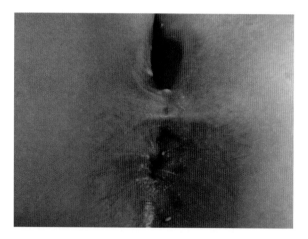

FIGURE 7.7.1   Eroded plaque with adjacent scarring: erosive lichen planus.

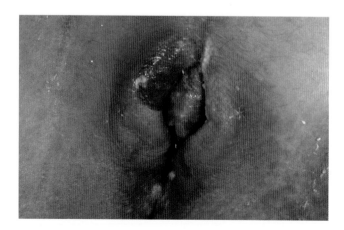

FIGURE 7.7.2   Erosive lichen planus.

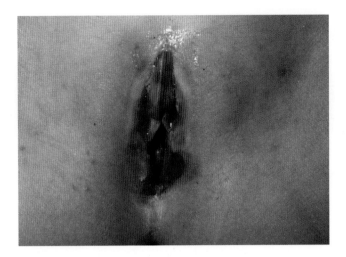

FIGURE 7.7.3   Erosive lichen planus.

Clinical course: If left untreated, architectural changes resulting in atrophy and scarring can follow, with loss of the labia minora, sealing of the clitoral hood, and burial of the clitoris. In the most severe cases, tissue destruction may lead to the development of synechiae and vaginal stenosis, which can result in hematocolpos, dyspareunia, and sexual impairment as a consequence of extensive atrophy and scarring with stenosis of the vaginal orifice. In long-standing, aggressive forms, possible malignant degeneration should also be taken into account, although this is still a controversial issue.

Diagnosis: It is suggested by the clinical features and supported by histological examination.

Differential diagnosis: Autoimmune bullous skin disorders (pemphigus vulgaris and bullous and cicatricial pemphigoid) may be ruled out by immunofluorescence studies. Bullous drug eruptions (fixed drug eruption and erythema multiforme) should also be considered.

Therapy: The management of erosive lichen planus may be very challenging. As it is a chronic complaint, topical and systemic treatment may be required intermittently or continuously over the long term. There are few treatment options and no definitive treatments. The first-line medical treatment is generally an ultra-potent topical corticosteroid ointment. There has been some interest in the use of topical calcineurin inhibitors. Surgical release of vulval and vaginal adhesions and scarring may be performed to manage urination difficulties and allow intercourse.

Bibliography

Cooper SM. Influence of treatment of erosive lichen planus of the vulva and its prognosis. *Arch Dermatol* 2006;142:289–94.

Helgesen AL, Gjersvik P, Jebsen P, Kirschner R, Tanbo T. Vaginal involvement in genital erosive lichen planus. *Acta Obstet Gynecol Scand* 2010;89:966–70.

Kennedy CM, Galask RP. Erosive lichen planus: Retrospective review of characteristics and outcomes in 113 patients seen in a vulvar speciality clinic. *J Reprod Med* 2007;52:43–7.

Lewis FM, Bogliatto F. Erosive vulval lichen planus—A diagnosis not to be missed: A clinical review. *Eur J Obstet Gynecol Reprod Biol* 2013;171:214–9.

Lotery HE, Galask RP. Erosive lichen planus of the vulva and vagina. *Obstet Gynecol* 2003;101:1121–5.

Simpson RC, Thomas KS, Leighton P, Murphy R. Diagnostic criteria for erosive lichen planus affecting the vulva: An international electronic-Delphi consensus exercise. *Br J Dermatol* 2013;169:337–43.

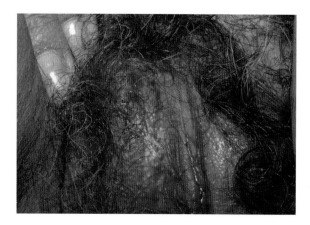

FIGURE 7.7.4   Single infiltrated and superficially ulcerated plaque: basal cell carcinoma.

7.7.2 Basal Cell Carcinoma

Clinical aspect: It may present as a single skin-colored, nonscaling, sometimes ulcerated papule or plaque that may be either asymptomatic or pruritic. It may sometimes have a very nonspecific and indolent clinical appearance, simulating a simple irritation, intertrigo, eczema, or psoriasis (Figure 7.7.4).

Definition: It is the most common type of malignant skin cancer, more often found on sun-exposed skin areas, but it occurs very rarely on the vulva.

Etiology: It is unknown. Several individual (fair skin, immune deficiency, nevoid basal cell carcinoma syndrome, and xeroderma pigmentosum) and environmental (ultraviolet light or ionizing radiation exposure, arsenic ingestion, previous trauma, chronic irritation, and syphilis) precipitating factors have been considered, although results have been inconclusive.

Epidemiology: It is rare, accounting for less than 5% of all vulvar neoplasms and less than 1% of all basal cell carcinomas, but vulvar involvement is reportedly four times more frequent than its male counterpart.

Clinical course: It grows locally at a slow rate. Metastases have occasionally been reported, especially in cases of the sclerosing type or with perineural invasion.

Diagnosis: It is usually made on histology.

Differential diagnosis: Dermal melanocytic nevus, seborrheic keratosis, neurofibroma, trichoepithelioma, sebaceous hyperplasia, dermatofibroma, acrochordon, wart, nodular melanoma, clear cell acanthoma, and appendageal tumors.

Therapy: Local excision is usually curative. Incomplete excision may result in local recurrence, so close long-term follow-up is necessary.

Bibliography

Blok JL, Reesink-Peters N, Diercks GF, Reyners AK, Terra JB. Vulvar basal cell carcinoma with destructive consequences. *Ned Tijdschr Geneeskd* 2012;156:A5391.

Elwood H, Kim J, Yemelyanova A, Ronnett BM, Taube JM. Basal cell carcinomas of the vulva: High-risk human papillomavirus DNA detection, p16 and BerEP4 expression. *Am J Surg Pathol* 2014;38:542–7.

Fleury AC, Junkins-Hopkins JM, Diaz-Montes T. Vulvar basal cell carcinoma in a 20-year-old: Case report and review of the literature. *Gynecol Oncol Case Rep* 2011;2:26–7.

Garg M, Sharma P, Gupta S, Sankhwar SN. Giant vulvar basal cell carcinoma. *BMJ Case Rep* 2013;2013:doi: 10.1136/bcr-2013-200180.

Jones ISC, Crandon A, Sanday K. Vulvar basal cell carcinoma: A retrospective study of 29 cases from Queensland. *Open J Obstet Gynecol* 2012;2:136–9.

Kara M, Colgecen E, Yildirim EN. Vulvar basal cell carcinoma. *Indian J Pathol Microbiol* 2012;55:583–4.

Mulvany NJ, Rayoo M, Allen DG. Basal cell carcinoma of the vulva: A case series. *Pathology* 2012;44:528–33.

7.7.3 Squamous Cell Carcinoma

Clinical aspect: The lesions are usually unifocal and approximately 1–2 cm in size. They appear as warty or ulcerated, variably colored (from white to red) papules or plaques that may occasionally bleed (Figures 7.7.5 and 7.7.6).

Definition: It is a malignant epithelial tumor originating from epidermal keratinocytes.

Etiology: Risk factors are advanced age, immunosuppression, and pre-existing conditions, such as high-risk HPV infections and long-standing lichen sclerosus or, less often, other chronic vulvar inflammatory disorders, such as lichen planus.

Epidemiology: It is a rare disease mainly seen in elderly women that accounts for 5% of all female genital malignancies.

Clinical course: Local invasion and lymphatic spread to inguinal lymph nodes is common.

Diagnosis: Biopsy is essential to rule out other conditions and identify the histological subtype.

Differential diagnosis: Verrucous carcinoma, hypertrophic lichen planus or lichen simplex chronicus, anogenital warts, and extramammary Paget disease.

Therapy: Staging is essential for proper treatment planning; whenever feasible, surgical excision is recommended.

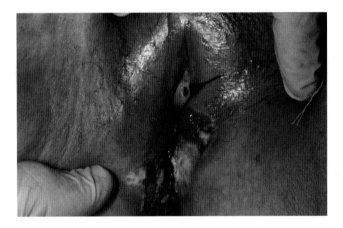

FIGURE 7.7.5   Indurated and eroded plaque: squamous cell carcinoma.

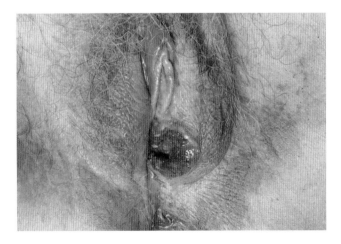

FIGURE 7.7.6   Raised and ulcerated plaque: squamous cell carcinoma.

Bibliography

Dittmer C, Fischer D, Diedrich K, Thill M. Diagnosis and treatment options of vulvar cancer: A review. *Arch Gynecol Obstet* 2012;285:183–93.

Nguessan KL, Mian DB, Kasse K, Boni S. Vulvar squamous cell carcinoma developing in a young black African HIV woman. *Eur J Gynaecol Oncol* 2013;34:496–9.

Reade CJ, Eiriksson LR, Mackay H. Systemic therapy in squamous cell carcinoma of the vulva: Current status and future directions. *Gynecol Oncol* 2014;132:780–9.

Sagdeo A, Gormley RH, Abuabara K, Tyring SK, Rady P, Elder DE, Kovarik CL. The diagnostic challenge of vulvar squamous cell carcinoma: Clinical manifestations and unusual human papillomavirus types. *J Am Acad Dermatol* 2014;70:586–8.

Stehman FB, Look KY. Carcinoma of the vulva. *Obstet Gynecol* 2006;107:719–33.

Tyring SK. Vulvar squamous cell carcinoma: Guidelines for early diagnosis and treatment. *Am J Obstet Gynecol* 2003;189:S17–23.

7.8 Sclerotic/Hypochromic Papules and/or Plaques

7.8.1 Lichen Sclerosus

Clinical aspect: Circumscribed, ivory white, smooth and shiny papules or plaques showing a fine superficial atrophic wrinkling ("cigarette-paper") that commonly start in the preclitoral area, spreading to involve the entire labia minora and interlabial sulcus and then extending down through the perineum and the perianal area, forming the typical keyhole or figure-8 pattern (Figures 7.8.1 through 7.8.4). Macular bruises and telangiectases may often be noted (Figures 7.8.5 and 7.8.6). Occasionally, hyperkeratosis (Figures 7.8.7 and 7.8.8) or erosions (Figure 7.8.9) may occur. It may sometimes be asymptomatic, but severe pruritus is generally present. Burning, soreness, pain, dyspareunia, dysuria, or bleeding may also occur.

Definition: It is a chronic mucocutaneous inflammatory disease that affects the genitalia and, less often, the extragenital skin (upper trunk and arms). Synonyms are hyperplastic dystrophy and kraurosis vulvae.

Etiology: Its cause is unknown. It is probably multifactorial and influenced by genetic (familial occurrence), immunological (association with autoimmune disorders), hormonal (higher prevalence in prepuberal girls, in postmenopausal women and in premenopausal women taking oral contraceptives),

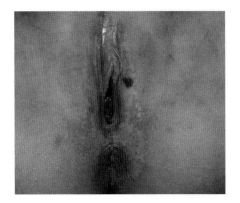

FIGURE 7.8.1 Lichen sclerosus with perineal involvement. A melanocytic nevus is also detectable.

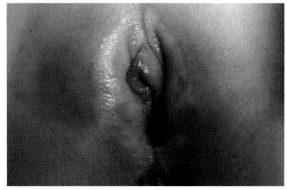

FIGURE 7.8.2 Lichen sclerosus with fine superficial atrophic wrinkling.

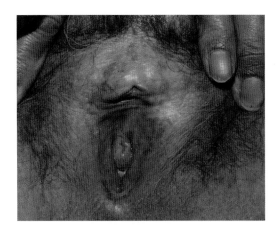

FIGURE 7.8.3 Vulvar flattening and constriction: lichen sclerosus.

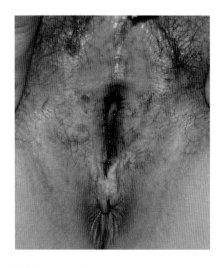

FIGURE 7.8.4 Fissuring and loss of normal vulvar anatomy: lichen sclerosus.

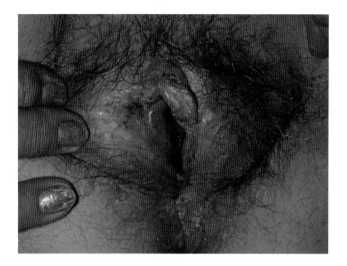

FIGURE 7.8.5 Lichen sclerosus with macular bruises.

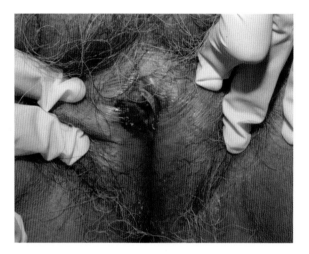

FIGURE 7.8.6 Lichen sclerosus with prominent macular bruises.

and local factors (triggered by traumas and chronic infections or irritation). The isomorphic (Koebner) phenomenon is described in this condition, with resultant lesions in old surgical scars, burn scars, sunburned areas, and areas subject to repeated trauma.

Epidemiology: The population rate is unknown. It is most common in middle-aged women (male:female ratio = 1:6), but can also occur in children (up to 15% of cases) from infancy onwards. Genital presentations outnumber extragenital reports by more than 5:1.

Clinical course: Over time, marked sclerosis may cause marked hypopigmentation, atrophy, and scarring with vulvar flattening, labial fusion, buried clitoris, constriction and fissures of the vaginal introitus, and loss of normal vulvar anatomy (kraurosis). This disabling disorder is often the cause of psychological discomfort as a result of sexual dysfunction, significantly impairing the quality of life. Risk of malignant degeneration is significant (3%–6% of cases) and should be suspected, prompting a skin biopsy, especially in case of persistent hyperkeratosis or erosions. It has been reported that prepubertal disease in girls may resolve spontaneously, although some of these patients may go on to suffer from various types of vulvodynia in adulthood.

Diagnosis: The clinical features are usually diagnostic. Histopathology may be performed in uncertain cases or to rule out malignancy.

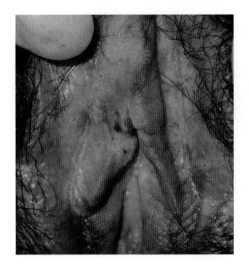

FIGURE 7.8.7 Lichen sclerosus with prominent hyperkeratosis.

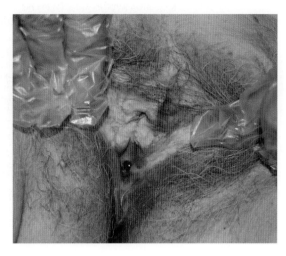

FIGURE 7.8.8 Lichen sclerosus with prominent hyperkeratosis.

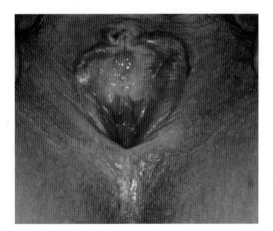

FIGURE 7.8.9 Lichen sclerosus with shallow erosions.

Differential diagnosis: Lichen planus, lichen simplex, vitiligo, postmenopausal atrophy, cicatricial pemphigoid, extramammary Paget disease, and sexual abuse.

Therapy: This disorder may be responsive to potent topical corticosteroids, although the patient should be warned that the clinical appearance does not always reverse, even if symptoms are relieved. Topical calcineurin inhibitors have been found to be helpful in some patients, but they do not work as rapidly or as effectively as potent topical corticosteroids, and deserve a role in maintenance treatment at best. Surveillance is recommended to promptly detect and treat any bacterial, mycotic, or viral superinfections that may result from protracted topical therapies. Mutilating gynecologic surgery for this benign disorder should be avoided, unless an associated malignancy is present.

Bibliography

Brodrick B, Belkin ZR, Goldstein AT. Influence of treatments on prognosis for vulvar lichen sclerosus: Facts and controversies. *Clin Dermatol* 2013;31:780–6.

Cooper SM, Ali I, Baldo M, Wojnarowska F. The association of lichen sclerosus and erosive lichen planus of the vulva with autoimmune disease: A case–control study. *Arch Dermatol* 2008;144:1432–5.

Doulaveri G, Armira K, Kouris A, Karypidis D, Potouridou I. Genital vulvar lichen sclerosus in monozygotic twin women: A case report and review of the literature. *Case Rep Dermatol* 2013;5:321–5.

Günthert AR, Faber M, Knappe G, Hellriegel S, Emons G. Early onset vulvar lichen sclerosus in premenopausal women and oral contraceptives. *Eur J Obstet Gynecol Reprod Biol* 2008;137:56–60.

Isaac R, Lyn M, Triggs N. Lichen sclerosus in the differential diagnosis of suspected child abuse cases. *Pediatr Emerg Care* 2007;23:482–5.

Virgili A, Borghi A, Toni G, Minghetti S, Corazza M. Prospective clinical and epidemiologic study of vulvar lichen sclerosus: Analysis of prevalence and severity of clinical features, together with historical and demographic associations. *Dermatology* 2014;228:145–51.

8

Plaques

Giuseppe Micali, Maria Letizia Musumeci, and Maria Rita Nasca

8.1 Red Plaques

8.1.1 Plasma Cell Vulvitis (Zoon)

Clinical aspect: It appears as single or multiple irregularly shaped and sharply marginated, fixed and not infiltrated, dark red, smooth and shiny plaques (Figure 8.1.1) that may sometimes show tiny brownish so-called "Cayenne pepper" spotting. Elective sites of involvement are the labia minora and majora, clitoris, fourchette, urethral meatus, and vaginal ostium. Multiple lesions are often bilateral and symmetrical and tend to join up progressively. Occasionally, ecchymotic, teleangiectatic, and purpuric patches or raised, granulomatous, nodular, or erosive plaques have been reported. This condition may be asymptomatic or be associated with pruritus, burning, pain, and dyspareunia.

Definition: It is a rare benign, circumscribed inflammation of the vulvar mucosa characterized by plasma cell infiltration. It represents the female counterpart of Zoon plasma cell balanitis.

Etiology: The specific cause of this condition is unknown. Suggested predisposing factors include warmth, friction, poor hygiene, herpes simplex, and other chronic infections.

Epidemiology: In contrast to plasma cell balanitis, it is an extremely rare skin condition (there have been only 31 cases reported worldwide). It is found in women ranging in age from 26 to 70 years and has never been observed in prepubertal girls.

Clinical course: It is chronic and relapsing, with lesions tending to persist for many years. Neoplastic progression has never been reported.

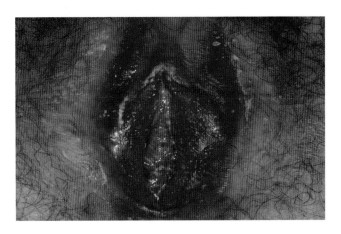

FIGURE 8.1.1 Sharply marginated, red and smooth plaques: plasma cell vulvitis.

Diagnosis: Skin biopsy is usually performed to confirm the clinical diagnosis.

Differential diagnosis: This condition must be primarily differentiated by erythroplasia. Common bacterial and fungal infections (candidiasis) should also be ruled out.

Therapy: Topical corticosteroids and intralesional injections have been used with varying degrees of success. Topical calcineurin inhibitors, retinoids, and interferon have shown some benefit in a few patients. Other therapies to consider include topical antifungals and antibiotics, caudal nerve blocks, cryotherapy, and simple excision.

Bibliography

Çelik A, Haliloglu B, Tanriöver Y, Ilter E, Gündüz T, Ulu I, Midi A, Özekici Ü. Plasma cell vulvitis: A vulvar itching dilemma. *Indian J Dermatol Venereol Leprol* 2012;78:230.

David L, Massey K. Plasma cell vulvitis and response to topical steroids: A case report. *Int J STD AIDS* 2003;14:568–9.

Fernández-Aceñero MJ, Córdova S. Zoon's vulvitis (vulvitis circumscripta plasmacellularis). *Arch Gynecol Obstet* 2010;282:351–2.

Hindle E, Yell J, Andrew S, Tasker M. Plasma cell vulvovaginitis—A further case. *J Obstet Gynaecol* 2006;26:382–3.

Virgili A, Mantovani L, Lauriola MM, Marzola A, Corazza M. Tacrolimus 0.1% ointment: Is it really effective in plasma cell vulvitis? Report of four cases. *Dermatology* 2008;216:243–6.

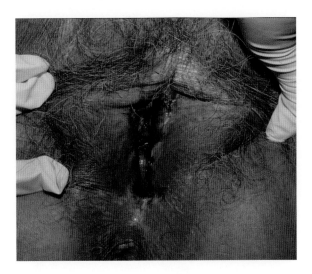

FIGURE 8.1.2   Dark red plaque surrounded by sclerotic changes: erythroplasia in a patient with lichen sclerosus.

8.1.2 Erythroplasia

Clinical aspect: It appears as single, fixed, slowly enlarging erythematous plaques, with clear-cut edges and a smooth, shiny surface (Figure 8.1.2). It is asymptomatic and is generally localized on the labia minora.

Definition: Erythroplasia of Queyrat is a premalignant condition of the visible mucous membranes and represents an intraepithelial squamous cell carcinoma (carcinoma *in situ*). In nonmucosal areas, carcinoma *in situ* is referred to as Bowen's disease.

Etiology: Poor hygiene and chronic irritation have been claimed to be possible risk factors, but its causes remain unknown.

Epidemiology: It is mostly observed in middle-aged women.

Clinical course: Erosions and ulceration may occur and usually reveal evolution into an invasive squamous cell carcinoma.

Diagnosis: It requires histopathological examination of a biopsy sample.

Differential diagnosis: The most important differential diagnosis is plasma cell vulvitis. Common bacterial and fungal infections (candidiasis) should also be ruled out.

Therapy: Lesion removal by surgical excision or other ablative means (Mohs surgery, electrocautery, laser therapy, or photodynamic therapy) and close follow-up are indicated.

Bibliography

Krüger-Corcoran D, Vandersee S, Stockfleth E. Precancerous tumors and carcinomas *in situ* of the skin. *Internist* 2013;54:671–82.

Zolis L, Shier M. Vulvar intraepithelial neoplasia (erythroplasia of Queyrat). *J Obstet Gynaecol Can* 2008;30:647–8.

8.1.3 Extramammary Paget Disease

Clinical aspect: The most common location is the vulva. Lesions often appear as diffuse erythematous, thickened, moist, and irregular scaling plaques similar to eczematous changes; less often, a crusting, eroded, or ulcerated, lichenified, or leukoplakic plaque may be observed (Figures 8.1.3 and 8.1.4). Patients frequently complain of pruritus, burning sensations, and pain in the affected site.

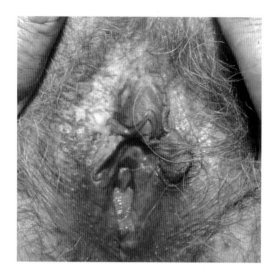

FIGURE 8.1.3   Thickened and lichenified leukoplakic plaque: extramammary Paget disease.

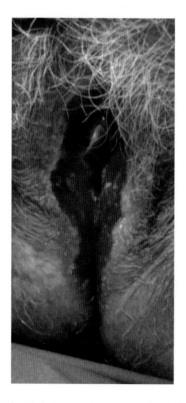

FIGURE 8.1.4   Erythematous, moist and eroded plaque: extramammary Paget disease.

Definition: Extramammary Paget disease is an uncommon intraepithelial adenocarcinoma that most commonly occurs in the anogenital region.

Etiology: It is thought to originate from intraepidermal apocrine glands or from pluripotent keratino-cyte stem cells as a result of an as-yet unknown multicentric carcinogenic stimulation.

Epidemiology: It is considered to be a relatively rare disorder, but its true incidence is unknown. It represents 1% of vulvar malignancies and occurs most frequently in postmenopausal women.

Clinical course: Untreated lesions progressively extend and persist for years before becoming invasive. Associations with underlying malignancies (genital, urinary, and gastrointestinal) have been reported. Recurrences are common, possibly because of its potential multicentric origin.

Diagnosis: The clinical diagnosis should always be confirmed by histopathology.

Differential diagnosis: Contact dermatitis and other eczematous conditions, common bacterial/fungal infections, Hailey–Hailey disease, psoriasis, lichen sclerosus, and squamous cell carcinoma.

Therapy: Radical surgical excision is usually effective. Other alternative options include Mohs surgery, CO_2 laser therapy, photodynamic therapy, or palliative radiation. Topical imiquimod has also been successfully used.

Bibliography

De Magnis A, Checcucci V, Catalano C, Corazzesi A, Pieralli A, Taddei G, Fambrini M. Vulvar Paget disease: A large single-centre experience on clinical presentation, surgical treatment, and long-term outcomes. *J Low Genit Tract Dis* 2013;17:104–10.

Edey KA, Allan E, Murdoch JB, Cooper S, Bryant A. Interventions for the treatment of Paget's disease of the vulva. *Cochrane Database Syst Rev* 2013;10:CD009245.

Kitagawa KH, Bogner P, Zeitouni NC. Photodynamic therapy with methyl-aminolevulinate for the treatment of double extrammamary Paget's disease. *Dermatol Surg* 2011:37:1043–6.

Villada G, Farooq U, Yu W, Diaz JP, Milikowski C. Extramammary Paget disease of the vulva with underlying mammary-like lobular carcinoma: A case report and review of the literature. *Am J Dermatopathol* 2014 [Epub ahead of print].

8.2 Scaling Plaques

8.2.1 Psoriasis

Clinical aspect: Although inverse psoriasis is the most common form of presentation in the vulvar area, isolated, thick, erythematous plaques covered with scales, sparing the mucosa, may also be observed (Figure 8.2.1). Psoriatic patches occurring on the vulva may sometimes show ill-defined edges or silvery–white adherent scales (Figure 8.2.2) or develop deep painful fissures (Figure 8.2.3). Mild or sometimes intense pruritus are often reported.

Definition: Psoriasis is a chronic and/or relapsing inflammatory skin disorder clinically presenting with erythematous patches covered by silver–white scales and typically occurring on the scalp, elbows, and knees.

Etiology: Koebner's phenomenon due to mechanical or chemical irritation likely plays a role in the onset of vulvar lesions.

Epidemiology: In most cases, genital psoriasis is part of a more generalized disease and occurs in up to 40% of patients with plaque psoriasis. Exclusive genital involvement is reported only in 2%–5% of psoriatic patients.

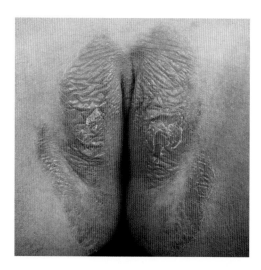

FIGURE 8.2.1   Symmetrical, thick, erythematous and scaling plaques with sharply defined edges: psoriasis.

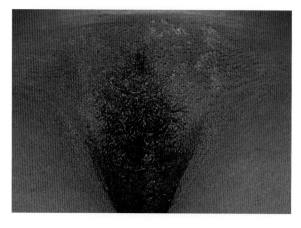

FIGURE 8.2.2   Multiple and coalescing plaques covered with silvery scales on the pubic area in a dark-skinned patient: psoriasis.

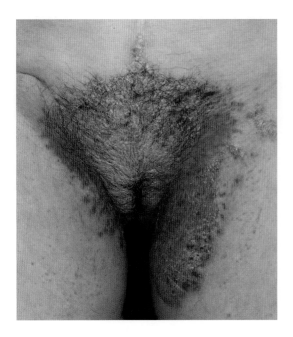

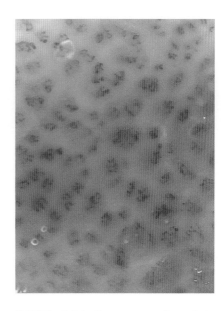

FIGURE 8.2.4 Dermoscopy of psoriasis: presence of dilated and tortuous capillaries with a "bushy" aspect.

FIGURE 8.2.3 Large erythematous and scaling plaque extending to the entire vulvoperineal area: psoriasis.

Clinical course: As a chronic and relapsing disorder, vulvar psoriasis may be stressful for patients, causing sexual concerns and considerably impairing their quality of life.

Diagnosis: The clinical diagnosis is not difficult when typical psoriatic patches are evident in the vulvar area or elsewhere. However, a skin biopsy may be necessary if other noninvasive diagnostic methods, such as videodermatoscopy, do not indicate the correct diagnosis, unequivocally showing at higher magnifications (×100–×400) dilated, elongated, and convoluted capillaries with a typical "glomerular" or "bushy" pattern (Figure 8.2.4). Microbiological investigations may be useful for ruling out primary or secondary infections.

Differential diagnosis: Fungal infections, eczema, and erythrasma.

Therapy: In case of exclusive genital involvement, topical corticosteroids, in combination or not with vitamin D analogs (calcipotriol), are indicated. Irritant topicals are better avoided, as they can worsen symptoms. Calcineurin inhibitors (pimecrolimus ointment or tacrolimus cream) may be an option. Systemic treatment is indicated when vulvar involvement occurs as part of a severe generalized psoriasis. Patients should be advised to follow accurate local hygiene measures to prevent bacterial and/or fungal secondary infections related to the disease itself or that are favored by the long-term use of topical steroids or immunomodulators.

Bibliography

Kapila S, Bradford J, Fischer G. Vulvar psoriasis in adults and children: A clinical audit of 194 cases and review of the literature. *J Low Genit Tract Dis* 2012;16:364–71.

Meeuwis KA, de Hullu JA, Massuger LF, van de Kerkhof PC, van Rossum MM. Genital psoriasis: A systematic literature review on this hidden skin disease. *Acta Derm Venereol* 2011;91:5–11.

Meeuwis KA, de Hullu JA, Van De Nieuwenhof HP, Evers AW, Massuger LF, van de Kerkhof PC, van Rossum MM. Quality of life and sexual health in patients with genital psoriasis. *Br J Dermatol* 2011;164:1247–55.

Meeuwis KA, van de Kerkhof PC, Massuger LF, de Hullu JA, van Rossum MM. Patients' experience of psoriasis in the genital area. *Dermatology* 2012;224:271–6.

Micali G, Lacarrubba F, Musumeci ML, Massimino D, Nasca MR. Cutaneous vascular patterns in psoriasis. *Int J Dermatol* 2010;49:249–56.

Zamirska A, Reich A, Berny-Moreno J, Salomon J, Szepietowski JC. Vulvar pruritus and burning sensation in women with psoriasis. *Acta Derm Venereol* 2008;88:132–5.

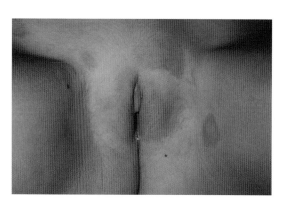

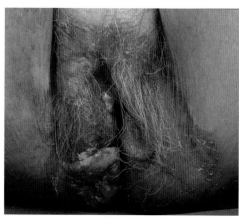

FIGURE 8.2.5 Well-defined patches with mild superficial wrinkling and scaling: parapsoriasis.

FIGURE 8.2.6 Thick and infiltrated erythematous plaque: T cell lymphoma.

8.2.2 T Cell Lymphoma

Clinical aspect: It may present with patches, plaques, tumors, ulcerations, or generalized erythema and can involve the lymph nodes and peripheral blood. Long-standing scaling plaques with a characteristic cigarette-paper appearance (parapsoriasis) (Figure 8.2.5) may precede the development of a frank T cell lymphoma (mycosis fungoides) (Figure 8.2.6).

Definition: Lymphomas are malignant proliferations of lymphocytes.

Etiology: It is unknown.

Epidemiology: It is usually observed in the elderly and is rare in infancy. Genital involvement may be primary or secondary. Primary lymphomas are extremely rare.

Clinical course: The outcome depends on the histological subtype, cytogenetics, and clinical features, but prognosis is unfavorable in the majority of cases.

Diagnosis: A skin biopsy is required to confirm the diagnosis. Molecular analysis of clonal T cell receptor γ gene rearrangements performed with PCR techniques is recommended. All patients should ideally be reviewed by an appropriate multidisciplinary team.

Differential diagnosis: T cell lymphomas may mimic: benign skin disorders, such as eczema (including contact dermatitis), psoriasis, lichen sclerosus, and pseudolymphoma; infections, such as secondary syphilis or coccidioidomycosis; and malignant tumors, such as carcinomas and malignant histiocytoses.

Therapy: Appropriate therapy depends upon a variety of factors, including the stage, the patient's overall health, the presence of symptoms, and patient-specific issues, such as cost of care and access to health care facilities. In general, therapies can be categorized as skin-directed (topical), phototherapeutic, and systemic treatments (chemotherapy).

Bibliography

Lagoo AS, Robboy SJ. Lymphoma of the female genital tract: Current status. *Int J Gynecol Pathol* 2006; 25:1–21.

Martorell M, Gaona Morales JJ, Garcia JA, Manuel Gutierrez Herrera J, Grau FG, Calabuig C, Vallés AP. Transformation of vulvar pseudolymphoma (lymphoma-like lesion) into a marginal zone B-cell lymphoma of labium majus. *J Obstet Gynaecol Res* 2008;34:699–705.

Zizi-Sermpetzoglou A, Petrakopoulou N, Tepelenis N, Savvaidou V, Vasilakaki T. Intravascular T-cell lymphoma of the vulva, CD30 positive: A case report. *Eur J Gynaecol Oncol* 2009;30:586–8.

8.3 Keratotic Plaques

8.3.1 Lichen Simplex Chronicus (Squamous Cell Hyperplasia)

Clinical aspect: It mostly affects the labia majora with one or more ill-defined, erythematous, grayish, scaling, thickened, hyperkeratotic plaques with prominent skin markings (Figures 8.3.1 through 8.3.4). Hyperpigmentation and varying degrees of overlying excoriation are usually evident. Itching is always present and may be severe, making this an extremely uncomfortable condition.

Definition: It is a benign, chronic, pruritic, inflammatory disorder. It is also known as neurodermatitis.

Etiology: It is an idiopathic condition resulting from the perpetuation of the itch–scratch–itch cycle, with consequent squamous cell hyperplasia. Associations with anxiety, depression, or a family or personal history of atopy have been reported.

Epidemiology: It commonly occurs after 30 years of age and its prevalence is 0.5%.

Clinical course: It has a chronic, prolonged course. Bacterial and/or fungal secondary infections may occur as a result of continuous scratching. Unfortunately, even with effective therapy, the probability of recurrence is great.

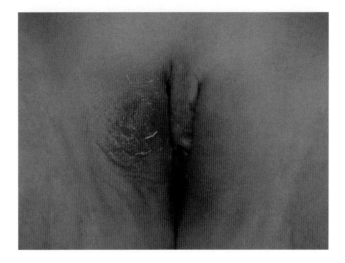

FIGURE 8.3.1   Ill-defined, erythematous scaling plaque: lichen simplex chronicus.

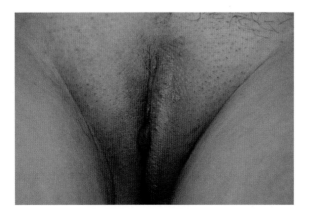

FIGURE 8.3.2   Infiltrated and erythematous plaque with prominent lichenification: lichen simplex chronicus.

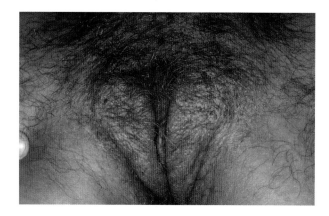

FIGURE 8.3.3   Lichen simplex chronicus with prominent scratching marks.

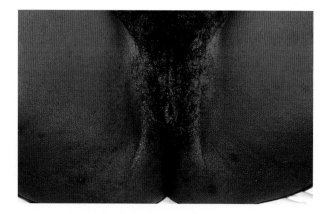

FIGURE 8.3.4   Lichen simplex chronicus in a dark-skinned patient.

Diagnosis: It is relatively simple with clinical examination. Biopsy is rarely necessary. Diagnostic workup includes skin swabs to rule out superinfections, patch testing to rule out allergic contact dermatitis, and a skin biopsy to rule out other chronic inflammatory skin conditions.

Differential diagnosis: Contact and atopic dermatitis, bacterial/fungal infections, lichen planus, psoriasis, lichen sclerosus, leukoplakia, Fox–Fordyce disease, epidermal nevus and verrucous, and squamous cell carcinoma.

Therapy: Moisturizers and corticosteroid ointments are indicated. Oral antihistamines may be used to control scratching. Antibiotics or antifungals should be used only if a documented bacterial or yeast superinfection occurs. Systemic corticosteroids or antidepressants should be reserved to selected cases.

Bibliography

Lichon V, Khachemoune A. Lichen simplex chronicus. *Dermatol Nurs* 2007;19:276.

Lynch PJ. Lichen simplex chronicus (atopic/neurodermatitis) of the anogenital region. *Dermatol Ther* 2004;17:8–19.

Rajalakshmi R, Thappa DM, Jaisankar TJ, Nath AK. Lichen simplex chronicus of anogenital region: A clinico–etiological study. *Indian J Dermatol Venereol Leprol* 2011;77:28–36.

Virgili A, Bacilieri S, Corazza M. Managing vulvar lichen simplex chronicus. *J Reprod Med* 2001;46:343–6.

8.3.2 Leukoplakia

Clinical aspect: It appears as single or multiple asymmetrical, ill-defined, whitish, thickened, and sometimes verrucous plaques usually located on the clitoris, labia minora, and inner aspects of the labia majora (Figures 8.3.5 through 8.3.7). Pruritus may be present and results in excoriations or fissurations with consequent soreness and pain.

Definition: It is a patch of mucosal squamous cell hyperplasia with prominent hyperkeratosis and is considered to be a precancerous condition.

Etiology: The roles of poor genital hygiene, chronic irritation, and oncogenic human papillomavirus (HPV) infection are still debated.

Epidemiology: There are no reliable data available.

Clinical course: Large lesions may cause vaginal orifice stenosis. If left untreated, evolution towards an invasive squamous cell carcinoma may occur. Malignant degeneration is clinically heralded by ulceration and/or bleeding.

Diagnosis: The clinical diagnosis must be confirmed by the histopathological examination.

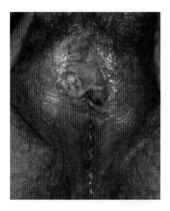

FIGURE 8.3.5 Asymmetrical, ill-defined whitish and thickened plaque: leukoplakia.

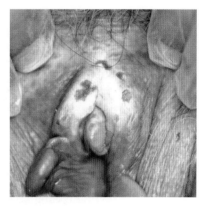

FIGURE 8.3.6 Large, infiltrated, partly eroded whitish plaque: leukoplakia.

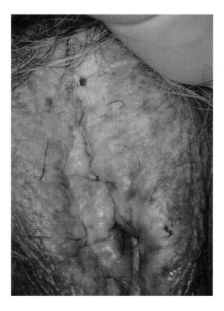

FIGURE 8.3.7 Grayish and thickened plaque with warty surface: leukoplakia.

Differential diagnosis: Lichen planus, lichen sclerosus, lichen simplex chronicus, psoriasis, chronic eczematous dermatitis, anogenital warts, and squamous cell carcinoma.

Therapy: The lesion should be removed by surgical excision, electrocautery, or CO_2 laser treatment.

Bibliography

Carter JS, Downs LS Jr. Vulvar and vaginal cancer. *Obstet Gynecol Clin North Am* 2012;39:213–31.

Dehen L, Schwob E, Pascal F. Cancers of the oral and genital mucosa. *Rev Prat* 2013;63:907–12.

Olek-Hrab K, Jenerowicz D, Osmola-Mańkowska A, Polańska A, Teresiak-Mikołajczak E, Silny W, Adamski Z. Selected vulvar dermatoses. *Ginekol* Pol 2013;84:959–65.

Skapa P, Robová H, Rob L, Zámečník J. Review of precancerous vulvar lesions. *Cesk Patol* 2012;48:15–21.

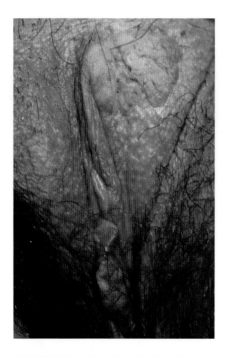

FIGURE 8.3.8 Raised and infiltrated plaque: Bowen's disease.

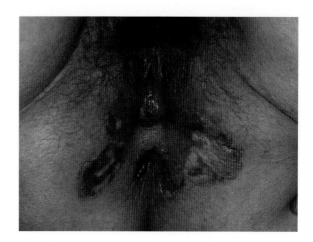

FIGURE 8.3.9 Thickened and ulcerated plaque: Bowen's disease.

8.3.3 Bowen's Disease

Clinical aspect: It may occur on vulvar skin as an asymptomatic, slowly enlarging, erythematous or brownish, often scaling, slightly infiltrated and sometimes ulcerated plaque of variable size and with irregular edges (Figures 8.3.8 and 8.3.9).

Definition: It is a cutaneous precancerous condition (*in situ* squamous cell carcinoma).

Etiology: Generic risk factors are exposure to chemical (arsenic) or physical (ultraviolet light and x-rays) carcinogens and HPV infections.

Epidemiology: It is not exceedingly rare. Its incidence increases with advancing age.

Clinical course: If left untreated, it invariably progresses towards an invasive squamous cell carcinoma.

Diagnosis: It is based on histopathological examination.

Differential diagnosis: Bowenoid papulosis, seborrheic keratosis, and pigmented basal cell carcinoma.

Therapy: Treatment options include surgical excision, cryotherapy, electrocautery, and photodynamic therapy.

Bibliography

Kutlubay Z, Engin B, Zara T, Tüzün Y. Anogenital malignancies and premalignancies: Facts and controversies. *Clin Dermatol* 2013;31:362–73.

Sheen YS, Sheen YT, Sheu HM, Sheen MC. Bowen disease of the vulva successfully treated with intraarterial infusion chemotherapy. *J Am Acad Dermatol* 2013;69:e305–6.

Yuan GW, Wu LY, Zhang R, Li XG. Clinical analysis for 18 cases of vulvar Bowen's disease. *Zhonghua Fu Chan Ke Za Zhi* 2013;48:925–8.

9

Nodules

Pompeo Donofrio, Franco Dinotta, and Giuseppe Micali

9.1 Nodules

9.1.1 Primary Syphilis (Chancre)

Clinical aspect: Approximately 3 weeks (incubation may range from 3 to 90 days) after the initial exposure, a chancre appears at the spirochetal portal of entry, mainly corresponding to the vulva or cervix in females. In 10% of cases, extragenital sites (including the anus, oropharynx, tongue, nipples, and fingers) may be affected. This is classically a single, reddish, firm, often eroded, painless and nonitchy nodule, with a clean base and sharp borders, between 0.3 and 3 cm in size (Figures 9.1.1 through 9.1.4). The chancre may sometimes show a central deeper ulceration with slightly elevated edges or be multiple in some patients. It may go unnoticed if it occurs in the inner part of the vagina or at the cervix. This lesion is highly infectious, oozing a serum that is rich in vital spirochetal organisms. Coexistent regional lymphadenopathy is typical. Inguinal adenitis is usually unilateral or, less often, bilateral, discrete, firm, mobile, and painless, without overlying skin changes.

Definition: Syphilis is a sexually transmitted disease that predominantly affects the genital area and is characterized by different clinical stages. Primary syphilis is the first disease stage and is marked by the development of a mucosal or skin lesion called a chancre.

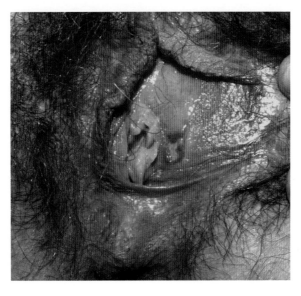

FIGURE 9.1.1 Single, sharply defined, reddish, firm and eroded nodule: chancre (primary syphilis).

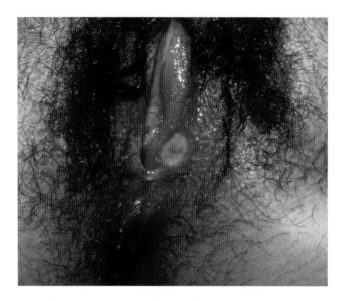

FIGURE 9.1.2   Firm nodule with sharp edges and shallow central ulceration: primary syphilis.

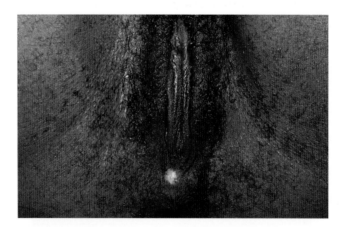

FIGURE 9.1.3   Primary syphilis in a dark-skinned patient.

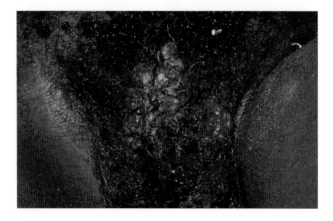

FIGURE 9.1.4   Primary syphilis in a dark-skinned patient.

Etiology: Primary syphilis is typically acquired by direct contact during intercourse with a sexual partner infected with *Treponema pallidum.*

Epidemiology: Syphilis is diffused worldwide, with highest rates in many developing countries (South and South-East Asia, sub-Saharan Africa, Latin America, and Eastern Europe). In recent years, its incidence has been rising in the Western world, especially in metropolitan areas and among homosexual men. The disease might be underestimated in women because genital primary lesions often go unnoticed.

Clinical course: Both the chancre and the reactive inguinal adenopathy clear in approximately 1 month (within 4–8 weeks), with or without therapy, usually with no scarring.

Diagnosis: Dark-field microscopy examination of serous fluid from the chancre may yield an immediate diagnosis. PCR is particularly suitable for extragenital locations, as it can also be performed on skin specimens. Anticorpal responses against infection may be detected by serologic testing, which, in the initial stages, is best performed using non treponemal VDRL and RPR tests. A treponemal test, such as treponema pallidum hemagglutination test (TPHA) or fluorescent treponemal antibody-absorption test (FTA-ABS), is recommended to rule out false-positive responses.

Differential diagnosis: Herpetic ulcers (especially chronic mucocutaneous anogenital herpes occurring with HIV infection), chancroid, lymphogranuloma venereum, and granuloma inguinale.

Therapy: Penicillin is the treatment of choice for syphilis. Doxycycline and tetracycline are alternative choices in case of penicillin allergy; however, due to the risk of birth defects, these are not recommended for pregnant women, who, if allergic to penicillins, may be treated with erythromycin. Antibiotic resistance has developed to a number of agents, including macrolides, clindamycin, and rifampin. Ceftriaxone may be as effective as penicillin-based treatments.

Bibliography

Braun J, Schäfer SD. Lesions of the vulva, fever, chills. You can expect to make this diagnosis more frequently again. Primary syphilis. *MMW Fortschr Med* 2013;155:5.

Dupin N, Farhi D. Syphilis. *Presse Med* 2013;42:446–53.

Mattei PL, Beachkofsky TM, Gilson RT, Wisco OJ. Syphilis: A reemerging infection. *Am Fam Physician* 2012;86:433–40.

Prabhakar P, Narayanan P, Deshpande GR, Das A, Neilsen G, Mehendale S, Risbud A. Genital ulcer disease in India: Etiologies and performance of current syndrome guidelines. *Sex Transm Dis* 2012;39:906–10.

9.1.2 Nodular Scabies

Clinical aspect: Reddish nodules correspond to lesions healing with development of an inflammatory granulomatous reaction (Figure 9.1.5). Itching is particularly intense, especially at night. Scratch marks and pathognomonic burrows (cunicula) on the vulva and elsewhere on the body (flexor aspects of the wrists, interdigital web spaces of the hands, dorsal feet, axillae, elbows, waist, and buttocks) may also be observed.

Definition: Scabies is a highly contagious cutaneous ectoparasitosis.

Etiology: It is caused by the mite *Sarcoptes scabiei hominis.*

Epidemiology: It is very common and diffused worldwide.

Clinical course: With proper diagnosis and treatment, the prognosis is good.

Diagnosis: Diagnosis is confirmed by the detection of the mites (Figure 9.1.6) or their eggs by *in vivo* dermoscopy or by light microscopic examination of skin scrapings.

Differential diagnosis: The differential diagnosis may include several other pruritic skin disorders.

Therapy: Topical antiscabietics are the mainstay of treatment.

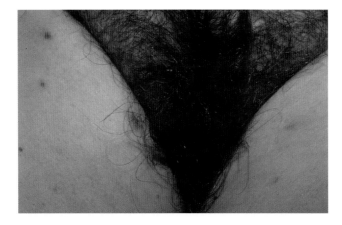

FIGURE 9.1.5　Multiple reddish itchy nodules: nodular scabies.

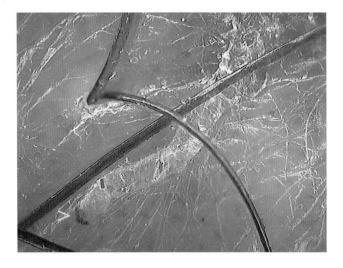

FIGURE 9.1.6　Dermoscopy of scabies: presence of the mite (arrowhead) at the end of a burrow, with a characteristic jet-plane or hang-glider appearance.

Bibliography

Czeschik JC, Huptas L, Schadendorf D, Hillen U. Nodular scabies: Hypersensitivity reaction or infection? *J Dtsch Dermatol Ges* 2011;9:840–1.

Moberg SA, Löwhagen GB, Hersle KS. An epidemic of scabies with unusual features and treatment resistance in a nursing home. *J Am Acad Dermatol* 1984;11:242–4.

9.1.3 Acrochordon (Fibroepithelial Polyp)

Clinical aspect: These lesions may be single or, more often, multiple nodules, ranging in size from 0.2 to 1.5 cm. They generally appear in the groin on healthy skin as skin-colored or hyperpigmented, pedunculated, soft and fleshy masses with a smooth or papillomatous surface (Figures 9.1.7 and 9.1.8). They are generally asymptomatic, but can become painful in case of inflammation secondary to traumatic ischemia.

Definition: It is a pedunculated skin tag that can be found in moist areas that are subject to irritation, such as the inguinal folds, the axillae, and the neck. Histologically, it is a benign fibroepithelial polyp made of lax fibrous tissue.

Etiology: The etiology is unknown.

Epidemiology: It is very common, especially in obese and/or diabetic patients. Prevalence increases with advancing age.

Clinical course: These lesions often increase in number and size with time, but remain benign. After torsion around the peduncle, they may become swollen, darker, painful, and undergo necrosis.

Diagnosis: It is clinical.

Differential diagnosis: Melanocytic nevus, neurofibroma, molluscum contagiosum, and neuroma.

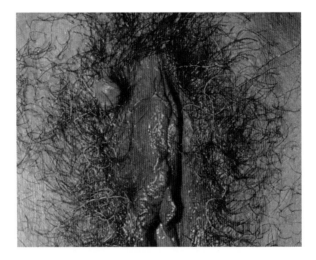

FIGURE 9.1.7   Solitary, raised, pedunculated, soft and smooth nodule: fibroepithelial polyp.

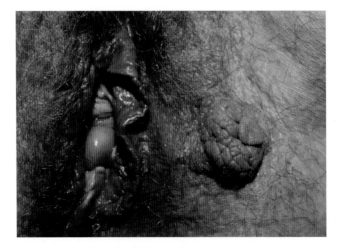

FIGURE 9.1.8   Large fleshy sessile nodule with papillomatous and cerebriform aspect: fibroepithelial polyp.

Therapy: Treatment is recommended only for symptomatic lesions or for aesthetic and/or functional reasons. Small, penduculated lesions may be removed with curved or serrated blade scissors, while larger skin tags may require simple excision. Other options are electrodesiccation, cryotherapy, and CO_2 laser ablation.

Bibliography

Ahmed S, Khan AK, Hasan M, Jamal AB. A huge acrochordon in labia majora—An unusual presentation. *Bangladesh Med Res Counc Bull* 2011;37:110–1.

Kassinove A, Raam R. Acrochordon of the labia. *J Emerg Med* 2013;44:e361–2.

Singh N, Thappa DM, Jaisankar TJ, Habeebullah S. Pattern of non-venereal dermatoses of female external genitalia in South India. *Dermatol Online J* 2008;14:1.

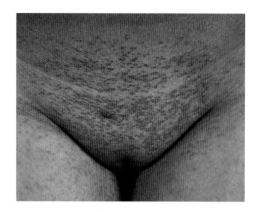

FIGURE 9.1.9   Multiple brownish papules and nodules scattered on the pubic area: syringomas.

9.1.4 Syringoma

Clinical aspect: Lesions are usually multiple and bilaterally distributed over the labia majora as small, skin-colored or yellowish-to-brownish papules or nodules (Figure 9.1.9). Pruritus is often reported. A third of patients also show syringomas on the eyelids.

  Definition: It is a benign eccrine sweat gland tumor.

  Etiology: The etiology is unknown.

  Epidemiology: Vulvar syringoma without extragenital involvement is extremely rare.

  Clinical course: It is uneventful.

  Diagnosis: Clinical suspicion and histopathological examination provide the diagnosis.

  Differential diagnosis: Any multicentric papular lesion of the vulva, especially if pruritic or painful, should be considered in the differential diagnosis.

  Therapy: Reported effective treatment options for vulvar syringomas include CO_2 laser treatment, cryotherapy, electrosurgery, and simple excision.

Bibliography

Akoglu G, Ibiloglu I, Durmazlar N. Vulvar nonclear cell syringoma associated with pruritus and diabetes mellitus. *Case Rep Dermatol Med* 2013;2013:418794.

Bal N, Aslan E, Kayaselcuk F, Tarim E, Tuncer I. Vulvar syringoma aggravated by pregnancy. *Pathol Oncol Res* 2003;9:196–7.

Dereli T, Turk BG, Kazandi AC. Syringomas of the vulva. *Int J Gynecol Obstet* 2007;99:65–6.

Garman M, Metry D. Vulvar syringomas in a 9-year-old child with review of the literature. *Pediatr Dermatol* 2006;23:369–72.

Huang YH, Chuang YH, Kuo TT, Yang LC, Hong HS. Vulvar syringoma: A clinicopathologic and immunohistologic study of 18 patients and results of treatment. *J Am Acad Dermatol* 2003;48:735–9.

Yorganci A, Kale A, Dunder I, Ensari A, Sertcelik A. Vulvar syringoma showing progesterone receptor positivity. *BJOG* 2000;107:292–4.

9.1.5 Fibroma, Fibromyoma, Dermatofibroma, and Angiofibroma

Clinical aspect: They usually appear as solitary, slightly raised, sessile or pedunculated, gray–brown, skin-colored or pigmented, mobile and indurated nodules (0.1–1 cm in diameter) with a smooth or papillomatous surface (Figures 9.1.10 through 9.1.12), often developing along the insertion of the round ligament into the labia majora. In dermatofibromas, lateral compression produces a slight indentation known as the dimple sign, which is characteristic of these tumors. Angiofibromas usually show a reddish hue.

Definition: They are benign solid connective tissue tumors.

Etiology: It is unknown.

Epidemiology: These lesions often occur in skin folds and are considered to be the most common benign vulvar tumors. They are usually observed in middle- and old-aged people.

Clinical course: These lesions usually cause no symptoms until they reach a larger size and/or are located near the introitus or urethra.

Diagnosis: The clinical appearance is sufficient for diagnosis.

Differential diagnosis: Dermal melanocytic nevus, histiocytoma, leiomyoma, neurofibroma, and keloid.

Therapy: As these are benign lesions, a specific therapy is not needed, but they can be removed for aesthetic and/or functional reasons by surgery, cryotherapy, cauterization, or laser therapy.

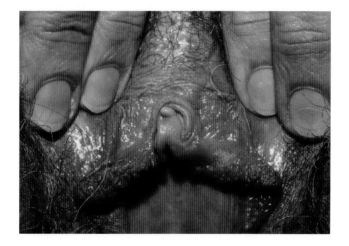

FIGURE 9.1.10   Skin-colored, elongated and indurated nodule: fibroma.

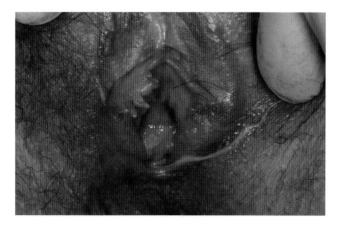

FIGURE 9.1.11   Raised, skin-colored papillomatous lesions: multiple fibromas.

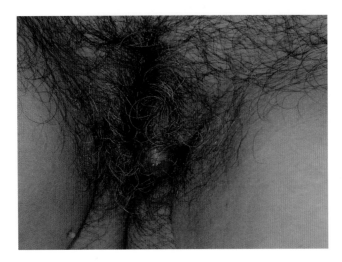

FIGURE 9.1.12   Solitary, raised, reddish nodule: angiofibroma.

Bibliography

Arsenovic NN, Abdulla K, Terzic M, Reed M. Synchronous presence of cellular angiofibroma and lipoma in vulvoinguinal region: A unique case report. *Am J Dermatopathol* 2009;31:468–71.

Dai LP, Zhao S, Yan CB. Cellular angiofibroma of vulva: Report of a case. *Zhonghua Bing Li Xue Za Zhi* 2009;38:847–8.

Isoda H, Kurokawa H, Kuroda M, Asakura T, Akai M, Sawada S, Nakagawa M, Shikata N. Fibroma of the vulva. *Comput Med Imaging Graph* 2002;26:139–42.

Kamble SN, Sambarey PW. Benign fibrous histiocytoma of vulva: Rare case. *J Obstet Gynaecol India* 2012;62:85–6.

Liu X, Ma YQ, Wang J. Prepubertal-type vulva fibroma: A clinicopathological study of two cases. *Zhonghua Bing Li Xue Za Zhi* 2010;39:40–3.

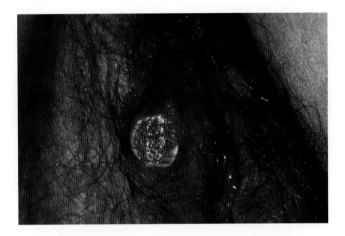

FIGURE 9.1.13   Rounded brownish nodule: hydradenoma papilliferum.

9.1.6 Hydradenoma Papilliferum

Clinical aspect: The tumor, which is nearly 1 cm in size, usually appears as a painless, soft, mobile, skin-colored or brownish nodule that is usually located on the labia majora (Figure 9.1.13).

Definition: It is a benign cutaneous adnexal neoplasm occurring mainly in the anogenital region of adult women.

Etiology: It is an adenoma with apocrine differentiation of unknown cause.

Epidemiology: It is rare.

Clinical course: The clinical course shows relentless growth and rarely enlarges conspicuously. It may become ulcerated or infected. Malignant change is extremely rare.

Diagnosis: The diagnosis is made by biopsy.

Differential diagnosis: Syringocystadenoma papilliferum, adenocarcinoma, and vestibular mucous cyst.

Therapy: Treatment is not necessary if the tumor is asymptomatic; in case of a symptomatic lesion, surgery is recommended.

Bibliography

Duhan N, Kalra R, Singh S, Rajotia N. Hidradenoma papilliferum of the vulva: Case report and review of literature. *Arch Gynecol Obstet* 2011;284:1015–7.

Veeranna S, Vijaya. Solitary nodule over the labia majora. Hidradenoma papilliferum. *Indian J Dermatol Venereol Leprol* 2009;75:327–8.

Virgili A, Marzola A, Corazza M. Vulvar hidradenoma papilliferum. A review of 10.5 years' experience. *J Reprod Med* 2000;45:616–8.

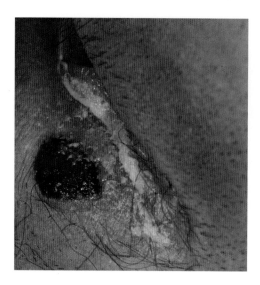

FIGURE 9.1.14   Deeply pigmented and indurated nodule: nodular melanoma.

9.1.7 Nodular Melanoma

Clinical aspect: It presents as a pigmented nodule, usually 0.5–1 cm in size, with rapid growth. It can be ulcerated and it can bleed easily (Figure 9.1.14).

Definition: It is a malignant tumor derived from melanocytes. Vaginal nodular melanoma is a rare form of noncutaneous melanoma.

Etiology: It is still unknown. Melanomas may develop in or near a previously existing precursor lesion or in healthy-appearing skin. Possible precursors of melanoma include common acquired nevi, dysplastic nevi, congenital nevi, and cellular blue nevi; however, in most cases, their risk of malignant transformation is low.

Epidemiology: It is rare, with incidence rates of approximately 0.1–0.2 per 1,000,000 women. The mean age of occurrence is 69 years (most common at approximately 60–70 years of age).

Clinical course: Lymph node status is the most powerful prognostic indicator for vulvar and cutaneous melanoma. Ulceration and tumor thickness of the primary lesion are the other important prognostic factors. It is associated with a very poor prognosis, as 5-year survival is rare.

Diagnosis: It is clinical and histopathologic.

Differential diagnosis: Melanocytic nevus, pigmented nodular basal cell carcinoma, bowenoid papulosis, seborrheic keratosis, pyogenic granuloma, and endometriosis.

Therapy: Complete surgical excision remains the treatment of choice. Sometimes, surgery is combined with chemotherapy.

Bibliography

Oiso N, Yoshida M, Kawara S, Kawada A. Amelanotic vulvar melanoma with intratumor histological heterogeneity. *J Dermatol* 2010;37:537–41.

Sharma R, Jain S. Nodular vulvar melanoma: A rare tumor with worse prognosis. *J Obstet Gynaecol India* 2012;62:87–8.

Virgili A, Zampino MR, Corazza M. Primary vulvar melanoma with satellite metastasis: Dermoscopic findings. *Dermatology* 2004;208:145–8.

10

Cysts

Francesco Lacarrubba, Ivano Luppino, and Maria Rita Nasca

10.1 Cysts

10.1.1 Vestibular Mucous Cyst

Clinical aspect: The classic presentation is an asymptomatic, smooth, shiny, sometimes bluish, dome-shaped, rounded cyst of up to 1 cm in diameter at the vaginal orifice or in the labia minora (Figures 10.1.1 and 10.1.2).

Definition: It is a simple cyst in the vulvar vestibule lined by mucus-secreting epithelium.

Etiology: It may be either the result of the obstruction of minor vestibular glands or derive from the urogenital sinus epithelium or mesonephric duct remnants.

Epidemiology: It is not uncommon. Mucous cysts are frequently discovered on routine pelvic examination.

Clinical course: It progressively enlarges, waxing and waning over several months. It may become sore and tender if infected. In addition, if very large, it may cause obstruction symptoms.

Diagnosis: It is clinical and histopathologic.

Differential diagnosis: Hidradenoma papilliferum, lipoma, fibroma, leiomyoma, and endometriosis.

Therapy: Treatment consists of simple excision and is recommended for symptomatic patients.

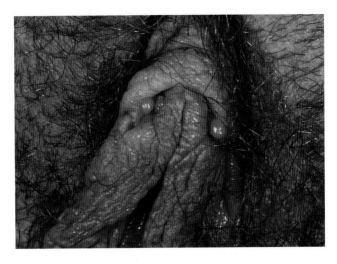

FIGURE 10.1.1　Multiple smooth, dome-shaped lesions: vestibular mucous cysts.

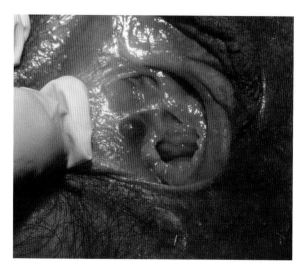

FIGURE 10.1.2   Purplish, rounded and shiny lesion: vestibular mucous cyst.

Bibliography

Hood AF, Lumadue J. Benign vulvar tumors. *Dermatol Clin* 1992;10:371–85.

10.1.2 Epidermal Inclusion Cyst

Clinical aspect: It is most commonly observed in the labia majora, but can also be found in the labia minora or elsewhere on the vulva as single or multiple, typically round, well-circumscribed, firm and mobile subcutaneous nodules, ranging in size from 2–3 mm to 1–2 cm (Figures 10.1.3 through 10.1.6). The overlying skin is smooth, yellowish and often shows an evident keratin-filled orifice.

Definition: It is a rounded structure filled with keratin debris, deriving from sequestration of proliferating benign epidermal or follicular keratinocytes within the outer skin layers, resulting in cyst formation and distension.

Etiology: It may be a late complication of traditional female genital surgery, a result of skin traumas, or a consequence of pilosebaceous duct obstruction.

Epidemiology: It is the most common genital cyst in women.

Clinical course: This lesion is asymptomatic unless rupture occurs. In such cases, superinfection ensues, and it may become very painful.

Diagnosis: Diagnosis is clinical and can be confirmed on biopsy.

Differential diagnosis: Hidradenoma papilliferum, lipoma, fibroma, leiomyoma, and endometriosis.

Therapy: Asymptomatic cysts need no treatment. Symptomatic cysts are surgically removed, but inflamed or infected cysts should not be excised and should receive prompt antibiotic treatment.

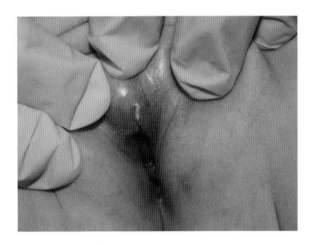

FIGURE 10.1.3   Single round mobile lesion in a newborn: epidermal inclusion cyst.

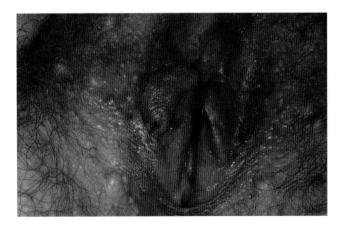

FIGURE 10.1.4   Multiple, scattered, smooth and yellowish nodules: epidermal inclusion cysts.

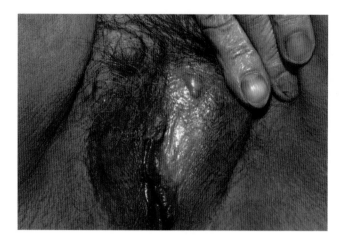

FIGURE 10.1.5   Epidermal inclusion cyst on the inner aspect of left labium majus.

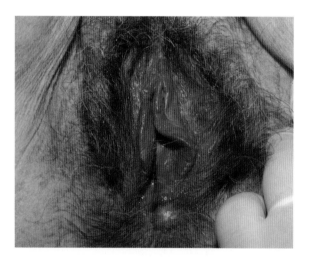

FIGURE 10.1.6   Smooth rounded cyst near the fourchette: epidermal inclusion cyst.

Bibliography

Apostolis CA, Von Bargen EC, DiSciullo AJ. Atypical presentation of a vaginal epithelial inclusion cyst. *J Minim Invasive Gynecol* 2012;19:654–7.

Hood AF, Lumadue J. Benign vulvar tumors. *Dermatol Clin* 1992;10:371–85.

Kondi-Pafiti A, Grapsa D, Papakonstantinou K, Kairi-Vassilatou E, Xasiakos D. Vaginal cysts: A common pathologic entity revisited. *Clin Exp Obstet Gynecol* 2008;35:41–4.

Kroll GL, Miller L. Vulvar epithelial inclusion cyst as a late complication of childhood female traditional genital surgery. *Am J Obstet Gynecol* 2000;183:509–10.

11

Ulcers

Pompeo Donofrio, Paola Donofrio, and Giuseppe Micali

11.1 Ulcers

11.1.1 Chancroid

Clinical aspect: The full-blown disease is characterized by an extremely painful ulcer that is 1–2 cm in diameter, with typically sharply defined, ragged, and undermined borders (Figure 11.1.1). The ulcers are often multiple, soft, covered by a grayish material, and may be shallow or deep. Inflammatory inguinal adenopathy is usually unilateral and occurs in approximately 50% of patients.

Definition: Chancroid is a sexually transmitted infection characterized by necrotizing genital ulceration, which may be accompanied by inguinal lymphadenitis.

Etiology: It is caused by *Haemophilus ducreyi*, a small, Gram-negative, facultative anaerobic bacillus, which is transmitted sexually by direct contact with purulent lesions.

Epidemiology: It is prevalent in Africa, the Caribbean basin and South-West Asia, and sporadically occurs in the developed world, usually associated with commercial sex work in metropolitan areas and related to individuals returning from endemic countries.

Clinical course: In its early stages, small tender inflammatory papules, soon turning into pustules, may be observed at the site of inoculation (vulva, cervix, and perianal area). Within days, these lesions may erode to form typical ulcers. Inguinal lymphadenitis develops within 1–2 weeks. Without treatment, ulcers may last weeks to months before undergoing self-healing.

Diagnosis: Combinations of clinical diagnosis and microbiological cultures are "gold standards" for the diagnosis of chancroid. When possible, every patient with chancroid should also be tested for other

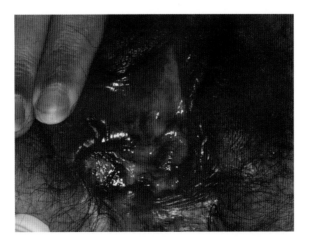

FIGURE 11.1.1   Soft and painful ulcer with undermined borders: chancroid.

common sexually transmitted diseases (STDs) (syphilis, genital herpes, gonorrhea, and chlamydia) and HIV.

Differential diagnosis: Lymphogranuloma venereum, granuloma inguinale, herpes simplex, and syphilis.

Therapy: Oral antibiotic treatment (erythromycin, azithromycin, ceftriaxone, and ciprofloxacin) is usually effective.

Bibliography

Hammond GW, Slutchuk M, Scatliff J, Sherman E, Wilt JC, Ronald AR. Epidemiologic, clinical, laboratory, and therapeutic features of an urban outbreak of chancroid in North America. *Rev Infect Dis* 1980;2: 867–79.

Kemp M, Christensen JJ, Lautenschlager S, Kemp M, Christensen JJ, Lautenschlager S, Vall-Mayans M, Moi H. European guideline for the management of chancroid, 2011. *Int J STD AIDS* 2011;22:241–4.

Lewis DA. Chancroid: Clinical manifestations, diagnosis, and management. *Sex Transm Infect* 2003;79:68–71.

Lewis DA. Diagnostic tests for chancroid. *Sex Transm Infect* 2000;76:137–41.

Roett MA, Mayor MT, Uduhiri KA. Diagnosis and management of genital ulcers. *Am Fam Physician* 2012;85:254–62.

Schmid GP. Treatment of chancroid, 1997. *Clin Infect Dis* 1999;28:S14–20.

11.1.2 Granuloma Inguinale

Clinical aspect: The clinical features may be variable, according to the disease stage. The initial lesion is a papule or nodule that arises at the site of inoculation from 8 days to 12 weeks after sexual contact with an infected partner. The most commonly affected sites in women are the labia minora, the pubis, the fourchette, and/or the cervix. These initial lesions are erythematous, soft and often pruritic, and eventually erode, leading to large, usually painless, foul-smelling, suppurative, "beefy red," and easily bleeding ulcers with clean, friable bases and distinct, raised, serpiginous and rolled edges (Figure 11.1.2). The ulcers, which are commonly observed in the skin folds, may be tender or painless, gradually enlarge centrifugally and develop subcutaneous granulomas, usually without lymph node involvement. Rarely, a proliferative reaction ensues with the formation of large, vegetating, hypertrophic, or verrucous masses, which may resemble genital warts. Dry ulcers may evolve into scarring plaques and be associated with lymphedema and swelling.

Definition: It is a chronic sexually transmitted disease that results in ulcerative, locally destructive lesions. Synonyms for granuloma inguinale are granuloma venereum and donovanosis.

Etiology: The causative agent is *Klebsiella granulomatis*, a Gram-negative pleomorphic bacillus, formerly known as *Calymmatobacterium granulomatis*, which is hypothesized to have low infectious capabilities because repeated exposure is often necessary for clinical infection to occur.

Epidemiology: This infection is endemic in tropical and subtropical areas (Western New Guinea, the Caribbean, Southern India, South Africa, South-East Asia, Australia, and Brazil), but very rare in temperate climates (Europe and North America). It is most commonly seen in sexually active people aged 20–40 years.

Clinical course: Secondary infection is common and increases patient discomfort. Abdominal visceral dissemination with fever, malaise, anemia, and weight loss may occur. In the late stages of the disease, lymphatic local damage, resulting in elephantiasis-like swelling of the external genitalia, is a frequent complication. An increased risk of squamous cell carcinoma development is also reported.

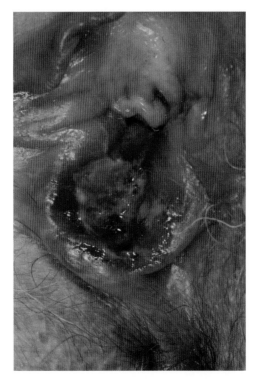

FIGURE 11.1.2   Large red, soft ulcer with rolled edges: granuloma inguinale. (Courtesy of Professor Marco Cusini).

Diagnosis: Diagnosis is clinical and confirmed by a tissue smear stained with Giemsa or Wright's stain showing intracytoplasmic Donovan bodies that look like safety-pins in mononuclear cells. Biopsy with Warthin–Starry silver stains and PCR methods can also be used.

Differential diagnosis: Chanchroid, lymphogranuloma venereum, herpes simplex, syphilis, and hidradenitis suppurativa.

Therapy: Oral antibiotics (erythromycin, azithromycin, streptomycin, tetracycline, or doxycycline) for at least 3 weeks or ampicillin for 12 weeks are standard treatments. Alternative treatments include trimethoprim–sulfamethoxazole and ciprofloxacin. Normally, the infection will begin to subside within 1 week of treatment, but the full treatment period must be followed in order to minimize the possibility of relapse.

Bibliography

Barroso LF, Wispelwey B. Donovanosis presenting as a pelvic mass mimicking ovarian cancer. *South Med J* 2009;102:104–5.

Bezerra SM, Jardim MM, Silva VB. Granuloma inguinale (donovanosis). *An Bras Dermatol* 2011;86:585–6.

O'Farrell N, Moi H; IUSTI/WHO European STD Guidelines Editorial Board. European guideline for the management of donovanosis, 2010. *Int J STD AIDS* 2010;21:609–10.

Roett MA, Mayor MT, Uduhiri KA. Diagnosis and management of genital ulcers. *Am Fam Physician* 2012;85:254–62.

Taneja S, Jena A, Tangri R, Sekhon R. Case report. MR appearance of cervical donovanosis mimicking carcinoma of the cervix. *Br J Radiol* 2008;81:e170–2.

Velho PE, Souza EM, Belda Junior W. Donovanosis. *Braz J Infect Dis* 2008;12:521–5.

11.1.3 Aphthosis and Behçet Disease

Clinical aspect: Vulvar lesions occur as single or multiple round or ovalar (diameter: 1 mm to 3 cm), well-defined and shallow ulcers, with a grayish fibrinous coating and raised, punched-out, erythematous edges (Figures 11.1.3 through 11.1.5). Similar to oral ulcers, vulvar aphthae are very painful; fever and malaise, sometimes reported in aphthosis, are the rule in Behçet disease (BD).

Definition: Aphthosis is a benign, chronic, and relapsing inflammatory condition characterized by single or multiple painful, self-healing canker sores on the oral or genital mucosa. Oral and genital lesions may coexist, and this condition is named aphthosis major or bipolar aphthosis. In BD, additional multisystemic symptoms due to the involvement of eyes (posterior uveitis), joints (arthritis and synovitis), and the central nervous system (meningoencephalitis) have also been observed; other manifestations include gastrointestinal involvement, cutaneous acneiform lesions, and thrombophlebitis.

Etiology: The cause is unknown. A pathogenetic role of the Th1-mediated immune response has been proposed. Genetic background and psychological factors have also been considered.

Epidemiology: Genital aphthosis is not as frequent as that of the oral mucosa, but precise epidemiologic data are unavailable. The incidence of BD has been estimated to be 0.2–1.0/100,000. BD is described in Europe and North America ("Western" BD) and in Japan ("Eastern" BD). "Western" BD is

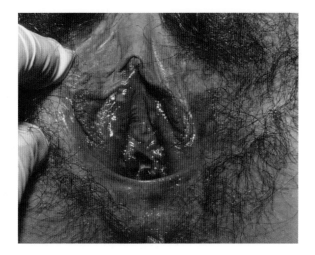

FIGURE 11.1.3   Shallow ulcers with fibrinous coating and raised sharply defined erythematous edges: aphthosis.

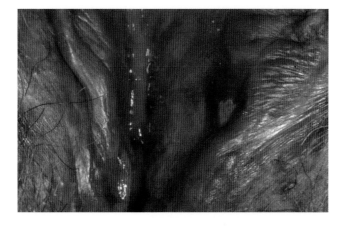

FIGURE 11.1.4   Whitish punched-out ulcer with surrounding erythema: aphthosis.

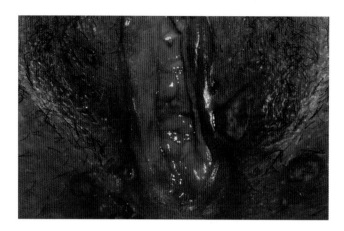

FIGURE 11.1.5   Multiple lesions: aphthosis.

more frequent in female patients and includes oral and genital ulceration and is less severe. "Eastern" BD is more frequent in male patients and it often presents as a central nervous system and ocular disorder.

Clinical course: The course is typically relapsing. Scarring is unusual, but high rates are reported in some series.

Diagnosis: Clinical features and past medical history usually provide the diagnosis, which for BD must also be supported by the fulfillment of the international diagnostic criteria.

Differential diagnosis: Herpes simplex, chancroid, granuloma inguinale, syphilis, lymphogranuloma venereum, Crohn's disease, tuberculosis, and idiopathic vulvar ulceration.

Therapy: Topical and systemic corticosteroids are the mainstay of treatment. Other medications that have been used for selected patients with refractory disease include colchicine, pentoxifylline, levamisole, dapsone, thalidomide, immune suppressors, and biologics.

Bibliography

Behçet H, Matteson EL. On relapsing, aphthous ulcers of the mouth, eye and genitalia caused by a virus. 1937. *Clin Exp Rheumatol* 2010;28:S2–5.

Hatemi G, Seyahi E, Fresko I, Hamuryudan V. Behçet's syndrome: A critical digest of the recent literature. *Clin Exp Rheumatol* 2012;30:S80–9.

Liu C, Zhou Z, Liu G, Wang Q, Chen J, Wang L, Zhou Y et al. Efficacy and safety of dexamethasone ointment on recurrent aphthous ulceration. *Am J Med* 2012;125:292–301.

Mohammad A, Mandl T, Sturfelt G, Segelmark M. Incidence, prevalence and clinical characteristics of Behcet's disease in southern Sweden. *Rheumatology* 2013;52:304–10.

O'Neill ID. Efficacy of tumour necrosis factor-α antagonists in aphthous ulceration: Review of published individual patient data. *J Eur Acad Dermatol Venereol* 2012;26:231–5.

11.1.4 Pyoderma Gangrenosum

Clinical aspect: Vulvar lesions are occasionally observed as deep, painful nodules or pustules (Figure 11.1.6) that break down very soon, draining a purulent discharge and forming an irregularly enlarging ulcer with undermined purplish borders, a necrotic base, and frequent satellite pustules.

Definition: It is a neutrophilic inflammatory dermatosis with distinctive clinical manifestations.

Etiology: The etiology is unknown, but probably involves altered immunity, as suggested by its frequent association with systemic autoimmune diseases (e.g., Crohn's disease, arthritis, and monoclonal gammopathy). Roles of defects in both humoral and cell-mediated immunological responses, as well as neutrophil dysfunction (impaired phagocytosis), have been proposed.

Epidemiology: It is found rarely on the vulva and very few cases have been described in the literature, most of which are associated with an underlying disease.

Clinical course: In 50% of cases, it is associated with an underlying systemic illness, particularly inflammatory bowel disease, polyarthritis, or myeloproliferative disorders.

Diagnosis: At present, the diagnosis is based on the clinical evaluation of the patient, as there is no diagnostic histopathological finding in this condition. Biopsy is therefore an essential step for the correct diagnosis and management of pyoderma gangrenosum.

Differential diagnosis: Bacterial and mycobacterial infections, chronic ulcerative herpes, tertiary syphilis, gangrene, tropical ulcers, and deep mycoses.

Therapy: The mainstay of treatment remains high-dose oral corticosteroids, although cyclosporine has also shown promising results. Other treatments that have been reported to show limited results include dapsone, sulfapyridine, sulfasalazine, clofazimine, azathioprine, cyclophosphamide, minocycline, intralesional steroids, chlorambucil, and hyperbaric oxygen. Topical tacrolimus and imiquimod represent interesting novel approaches to treatment. Surgical treatment in the form of debridement of the ulcer can exacerbate the condition and skin grafts are frequently rejected. Effective management of an underlying disorder often seems to result in improvement.

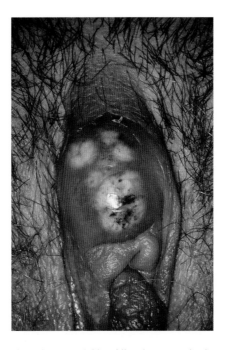

FIGURE 11.1.6 Painful collection of purulent material heralding deep necrotic ulceration: pyoderma gangrenosum.

Bibliography

Bhat RM. Management of pyoderma gangrenosum: An update. *Indian J Dermatol Venereol Leprol* 2004;70:329–35.

Borum ML, Cannava M, Myrie-Williams C. Refractory disfiguring vulvar pyoderma gangrenosum and Crohn's disease. *Dig Dis Sci* 1998;43:720–2.

Garcovich S, Gatto A, Ferrara P, Garcovich A. Vulvar pyoderma gangrenosum in a child. *Pediatr Dermatol* 2009;26:629–31.

Reed BG, Shippey S, Kremp A, Belin E. Vulvar pyoderma gangrenosum originating from a healed obstetric laceration. *Obstet Gynecol* 2013;122:452–5.

Sau M, Hill NC. Pyoderma gangrenosum of the vulva. *BJOG* 2001;108:1197–8.

Sripathi H, Rao R, Prabhu S, Singh M. Pyoderma gangrenosum affecting the vulva. *Indian J Dermatol Venereol Leprol* 2008;74:506–8.

Wiwanitkit V. Vulvar pyoderma gangrenosum. *Pediatr Dermatol* 2010;27:319.

12

Pigmentary Changes

Francesco Lacarrubba, Aurora Tedeschi, and Giuseppe Micali

12.1 Nonmelanotic Pigmentary Changes

12.1.1 Erythrasma

Clinical aspect: Progressively enlarging erythematous-to-brownish scaling patches arising in the inguinal folds and expanding in the vulvar area and inner thighs (Figure 12.1.1). The intergluteal cleft may also be affected. Friction and a warm and moist environment may favor maceration and the onset of pruritus, but most cases are asymptomatic.

Definition: It is a bacterial infection of the groin.

Etiology: Corynebacterium minutissimum is the causative agent. Predisposing factors include obesity, diabetes, a hot and humid climate, and profuse sweating.

Epidemiology: It is reported in all ages and in both sexes, but it is more frequent in young adults.

Clinical course: Relapses are frequent, especially in predisposed individuals.

Diagnosis: The clinical diagnosis may be confirmed by the typical red-coral fluorescence upon Wood's light examination. A skin swab is seldom necessary to rule out other conditions.

Differential diagnosis: Fungal infections, eczema, intertrigo, inverse psoriasis, seborrheic dermatitis, and acanthosis nigricans.

Therapy: Topical treatment with antibiotics (erythromycin or fusidic acid) is usually effective. Systemic treatment may be preferable in extensive or refractory cases.

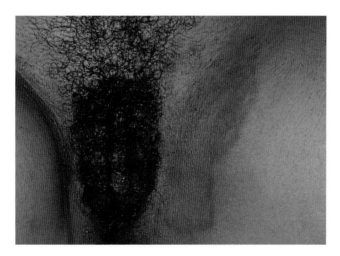

FIGURE 12.1.1 Patch of erythema and hyperpigmentation with sharp and slightly scaling edges on the left inguinocrural crease: erythrasma.

Bibliography

Chodkiewicz HM, Cohen PR. Erythrasma: Successful treatment after single-dose clarithromycin. *Int J Dermatol* 2013;52:516–8.

Laube S. Skin infections and ageing. *Ageing Res Rev* 2004;3:69–89.

Laufer B, Beckmann MW, Bender HG, Buslau U. Current diagnosis and therapy of inflammatory vulvar diseases. *Gynakologe* 1993;26:247–56.

Mattox TF, Rutgers J, Yoshimori RN, Bhatia NN. Nonfluorescent erythrasma of the vulva. *Obstet Gynecol* 1993;81:862–4.

12.1.2 Bruise/Purpura/Hematoma

Clinical aspect: They may present as purple or bluish streaks or lumps over the labia (Figures 12.1.2 through 12.1.4). They may be accompanied by vaginal bleeding.

Definition: Ecchymoses, contusions, and collections of partially clotted blood in the skin or mucosae.

Etiology: They usually follow a traumatic injury to the genital area. Straddle injuries are the most common accidental female genital traumas, defined as a fall in which the subject straddles an object compressing the soft tissue of the vulva between the object and the underlying bones of the pelvis.

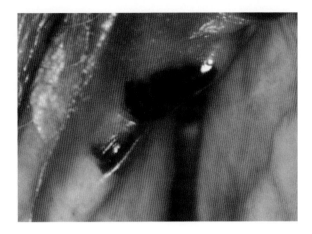

FIGURE 12.1.2   Detail of a bruise appearing as a bluish to black area of hyperpigmentation.

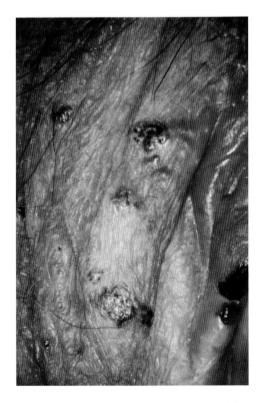

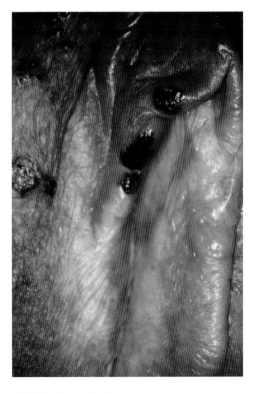

FIGURE 12.1.3 Multiple bruises resembling angiokeratomas.

FIGURE 12.1.4 Multiple bruises.

Epidemiology: The majority of reported cases occur between the ages of 2 and 6 years.

Clinical course: If hematoma occurs near the urethra, urination may be impaired.

Diagnosis: It is clinical.

Differential diagnosis: Bruising can sometimes be a sign of physical abuse or reveal a bleeding disorder or skin fragility. They may also mimic angiokeratomas.

Therapy: Small hematomas do not require any treatment. By contrast, in case of severe trauma, instrumental investigations and surgery may be necessary.

Bibliography

Dash S, Verghese J, Nizami DJ, Awasthi RT, Jaishi S, Sunil M. Severe haematoma of the vulva—A report of two cases and a clinical review. *Kathmandu Univ Med J (KUMJ)* 2006;4:228–31.

Machado-Linde F, Capel-Alemán A, Sánchez-Ferrer ML, Cascales-Campos P, Pérez-Carrión A, Ortiz-Vera C, Parrilla-Paricio JJ, Abad-Martínez L. Major post-traumatic non-obstetric large haematoma: Transarterial embolisation. *Eur J Obstet Gynecol Reprod Biol* 2011;154:118–9.

Okur MI, Yildirim AM, Köse R. Severe haematoma of the vulva and defloration caused by goring. *Eur J Obstet Gynecol Reprod Biol* 2005;119:250–2.

Virgili A, Bianchi A, Mollica G, Corazza M. Serious hematoma of the vulva from a bicycle accident. A case report. *J Reprod Med* 2000;45:662–4.

12.2 Melanotic Pigmentary Changes

12.2.1 Postinflammatory Hyperpigmentation

Clinical aspect: Macular patches that are often irregular with ill-defined margins, and show a sometimes uneven hyperpigmentation ranging from pale to deep brown (Figures 12.2.1 and 12.2.2).

Definition: It results from the accumulation of melanin in the dermis after an inflammatory process.

Etiology: It may be caused by drug intake (end stage of a fixed eruption) or other dermatological disorders localized to the vulva (e.g., lichen planus, discoid lupus erythematosus, and psoriasis).

Epidemiology: It is common.

Clinical course: It may take 6–12 months to fade, especially in dark-skinned subjects.

Diagnosis: It is clinical.

Differential diagnosis: Benign vulvar melanosis and vulvar intraepithelial neoplasia (*in situ* carcinoma or erythroplasia).

Therapy: The treatment tends to be difficult and long-lasting and is better avoided in the genital area.

Bibliography

Rock B. Pigmented lesions of the vulva. *Dermatol Clin* 1992;10:361–70.

Ronger-Savle S, Julien V, Duru G, Raudrant D, Dalle S, Thomas L. Features of pigmented vulval lesions on dermoscopy. *Br J Dermatol* 2011;164:54–61.

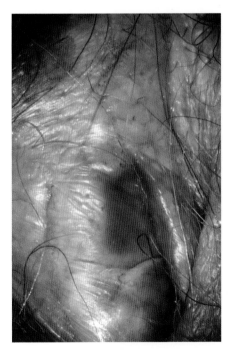

FIGURE 12.2.1 Reddish-brown macules with ill-defined margins: postinflammatory hyperpigmentation.

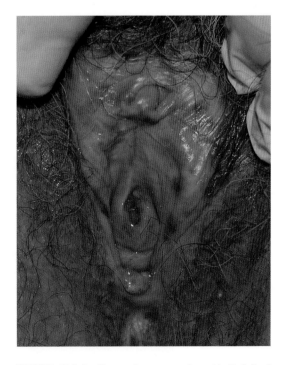

FIGURE 12.2.2 Uneven brown macules with ill-defined margins: postinflammatory hyperpigmentation.

12.2.2 Lentigo Simplex, Benign Vulvar Melanosis, and Lentiginosis

Clinical aspect: They may be found anywhere on the vulvar skin or mucosa as mottled or uniform dark brown to tan, smooth, pigmented macules with well-defined and sometimes jagged and irregular borders (Figures 12.2.3 through 12.2.8).

Definition: Hyperpigmented spots due to benign epidermal melanocytic hyperplasia of less than 4 mm in diameter (lentigo simplex) or larger (vulvar melanosis). Multiple lesions (lentiginosis) may sometimes occur in the setting of a congenital and/or inherited disorder (e.g., Peutz–Jeghers and LEOPARD syndromes or somatic mosaicism).

Etiology: They are due to melanin accumulation in basal keratinocytes and a slight increase in the number of normal melanocytes of unknown cause.

Epidemiology: They are more commonly seen in adults.

Clinical course: It is benign (atypia is uncommon). Lentigines can exist as isolated lesions or be associated with a spectrum of syndromes.

Diagnosis: It is based on clinical appearance. Videodermatoscopy may represent a useful noninvasive tool for both diagnosis and the follow-up of such lesions. When it is difficult to differentiate them from nevi or melanomas, histology is necessary. In case of large lesions, multiple biopsies may be necessary.

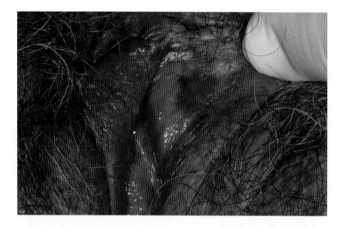

FIGURE 12.2.3 Uneven brown macules with jagged and irregular borders: lentigo simplex.

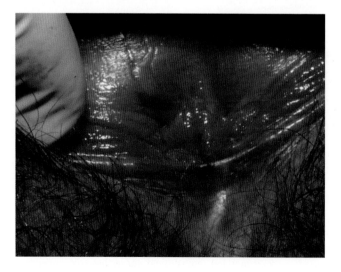

FIGURE 12.2.4 Smooth pigmented macule with sharply defined borders: lentigo simplex.

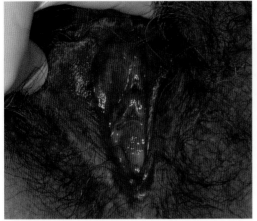

FIGURE 12.2.5   Benign vulvar melanosis.

FIGURE 12.2.6   Benign vulvar melanosis.

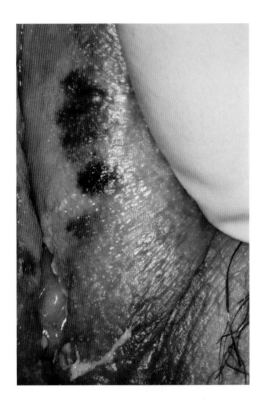

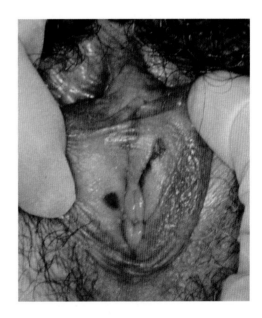

FIGURE 12.2.7   Benign vulvar melanosis.

FIGURE 12.2.8   Benign vulvar melanosis.

Differential diagnosis: Postinflammatory hyperpigmentation, melanocytic nevi, malignant melanoma, and pigmented basal cell carcinoma. In case of lentiginosis, it is important to rule out Peutz–Jeghers syndrome, LEOPARD syndrome, and inguinal freckling associated with neurofibromatosis.

Therapy: No treatment is recommended, but clinical surveillance is indicated. Excision should be prompt when clinically suggested.

Bibliography

Barnhill RL, Albert LS, Shama SK, Goldenhersh MA, Rhodes AR, Sober AJ. Genital lentiginosis: A clinical and histopathologic study. *J Am Acad Dermatol* 1990;22:453–60.

Ferrari A, Buccini P, Covello R, De Simone P, Silipo V, Mariani G, Eibenschutz L, Mariani L, Catricalà C. The ringlike pattern in vulvar melanosis: A new dermoscopic clue for diagnosis. *Arch Dermatol* 2008;144:1030–4.

Ferrari A, Zalaudek I, Argenziano G, Buccini P, De Simone P, Silipo V, Eibenschutz L et al. Dermoscopy of pigmented lesions of the vulva: A retrospective morphological study. *Dermatology* 2011;222:157–66.

Oliveira A, Lobo I, Selores M. Asymptomatic vulvar pigmentation. *Clin Exp Dermatol* 2011;36:921–2.

Rock B. Pigmented lesions of the vulva. *Dermatol Clin* 1992;10:361–70.

12.2.3 Junctional Melanocytic Nevus

Clinical aspect: Junctional melanocytic nevi appear as sharply marginated, hyperpigmented, tan to dark brown macules of variable size, but are usually small (Figures 12.2.9 through 12.2.11). Congenital melanocytic nevi appear as brown to dark macules that are commonly classified as small (<1.5 cm), intermediate (1.5–20 cm), or large/giant (>20 cm) (Figures 12.2.12 and 12.2.13).

Definition: Congenital or acquired benign proliferations and collections of melanocytes in small nests in the basal cell layer of the epidermis.

Etiology: It is unknown.

Epidemiology: They are observed on the vulva in approximately 0.1% of cases. Acquired junctional nevi appear in early childhood. Congenital nevi are observed at birth.

Clinical course: With time, junctional melanocytic nevi may become raised and verrucous, evolving towards a dermal melanocytic nevus. Pigmentation may fade progressively as a result of melanocytes settling deeper in the dermis.

Diagnosis: It is clinical, but may be aided by videodermatoscopy (Figure 12.2.14) or histology, which is indicated in uncertain cases to rule out other disorders.

Differential diagnosis: Lentigo, melanoma, seborrheic keratosis, and pigmented basal cell carcinoma.

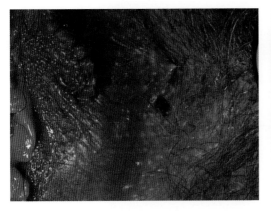

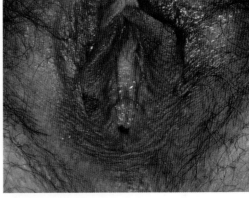

FIGURE 12.2.9 Small, sharply marginated, hyperpigmented macule: acquired junctional melanocytic nevus.

FIGURE 12.2.10 Acquired junctional melanocytic nevus.

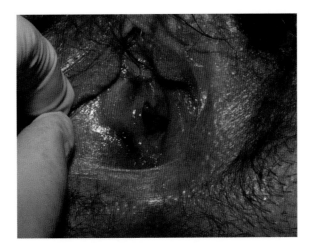

FIGURE 12.2.11 Acquired junctional melanocytic nevus.

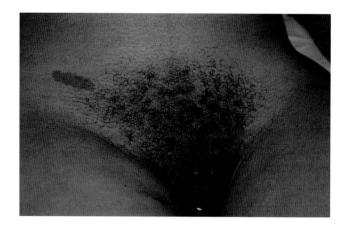

FIGURE 12.2.12   Congenital junctional melanocytic nevus.

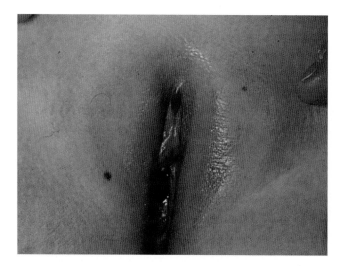

FIGURE 12.2.13   Congenital junctional melanocytic nevus on the right labium.

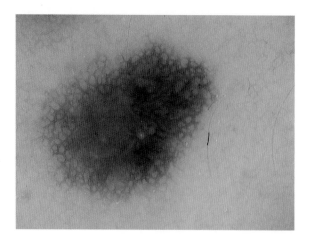

FIGURE 12.2.14   Dermoscopy of junctional melanocytic nevus: presence of regular brownish network of pigmentation.

Therapy: No treatment is necessary. Surgical excision may provide a diagnosis and a cure at the same time in case of diagnostic uncertainty. Nevi occurring on the vulva might be at higher risk for malignant degeneration; therefore, careful examination and follow-up is recommended.

Bibliography

Ribé A. Melanocytic lesions of the genital area with attention given to atypical genital nevi. *J Cutan Pathol* 2008;2:24–7.

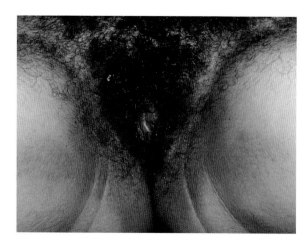

FIGURE 12.2.15   Symmetrical, poorly defined, velvety patches extending to the proximal medial thighs: acanthosis nigricans.

12.2.4 Acanthosis Nigricans

Clinical aspect: Symmetrical, brown, poorly demarcated, thickened patches that often appear velvety and prominently affect the crural creases, the hair-bearing surface of the vulva, the proximal medial thighs, the axillae, and the neck (Figure 12.2.15). This condition is usually asymptomatic, but some patients report local irritation and pruritus.

Definition: It is a diffuse pigmentary change occurring in intertriginous areas and skin folds and is often observed in obese or diabetic subjects.

Etiology: It is a common manifestation of insulin resistance. In addition to diabetes, it can occur in other endocrinopathies (hyperandrogenism). Other possible causes include underlying malignancies (most commonly, gastric adenocarcinoma; less frequently, endocrine, genitourinary and lung carcinomas, and melanoma) and medications (niacin, nicotinic acid, corticosteroids, estrogens, insulin, fusidic acid, protease inhibitors, and recombinant growth hormone).

Epidemiology: Because obesity is an ever-increasing problem, this condition is becoming more common as well.

Clinical course: Frequently, skin tags, which are an accentuation of the underlying papillomatous process, are found within the plaques. They tend to increase in size and number with time.

Diagnosis: It is made clinically by the symmetrical pattern of hyperpigmentation in skin folds and the velvety appearance. An underlying endocrinopathy or malignancy should be sought in patients who are thin and have no other evidence of insulin resistance.

Differential diagnosis: Erythrasma and intertrigo.

Therapy: It is not easily manageable. An essential step is the identification of the underlying cause because the treatment of the underlying disease leads to clearing of the cutaneous disorder. Weight reduction is the mainstay of treatment in most cases. Metformin as well as topical vitamin D analogs and oral and topical retinoids have been reported to be beneficial in some series, but results have been inconsistent.

Bibliography

Brickman WJ, Binns HJ, Jovanovic BD, Kolesky S, Mancini AJ, Metzger BE. Pediatric Practice Research Group. Acanthosis nigricans: A common finding in overweight youth. *Pediatr Dermatol* 2007;24:601–6.

Dubnov-Raz G, Weiss R, Raz R, Arieli R, Constantini NW. Acanthosis nigricans and truncal fat in overweight and obese children. *J Pediatr Endocrinol Metab* 2011;24:697–701.

Hermanns-Lê T, Scheen A, Piérard GE. Acanthosis nigricans associated with insulin resistance: Pathophysiology and management. *Am J Clin Dermatol* 2004;5:199–203.

Romo A, Benavides S. Treatment options in insulin resistance obesity-related acanthosis nigricans. *Ann Pharmacother* 2008;42:1090–4.

Valdés Rodríguez R, Moncada González B, Rivera Rodríguez SP, Aradillas García C, Hernández-Rodríguez H, Torres Álvarez B. Skin tags and acanthosis nigricans: Association with insulin resistance and overweight in Mexican children. *Gac Med Mex* 2011;147:297–302.

12.3 Hypochromic Pigmentary Changes

12.3.1 Vitiligo

Clinical aspect: Patients may present with vitiligo limited only to the genital area or show lesions elsewhere (back of hands, face, and extensor body areas subject to traumas). White nonatrophic amelanotic patches with normal skin markings and irregular but sharp edges may slowly and symmetrically enlarge, involving both the vulvar skin and the mucosae, often becoming confluent and reaching a considerable size (Figures 12.3.1 and 12.3.2). Hairs may or may not lose their pigmentation.

Definition: It is an acquired loss of pigmentation, probably on an autoimmune basis, characterized by circumscribed hypopigmented macules and patches.

Etiology: The etiology is multifactorial, with melanin pigment depletion likely resulting from immune-mediated melanocyte damage, as suggested by its frequent association with other autoimmune disorders (Hashimoto's thyroiditis, Graves' disease, Addison's disease, diabetes mellitus, alopecia areata, pernicious anemia, inflammatory bowel disease, and psoriasis). Genetic factors are also considered to play a role.

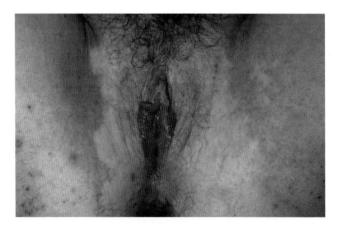

FIGURE 12.3.1   Achromic and sharply defined patches with jagged borders: vitiligo.

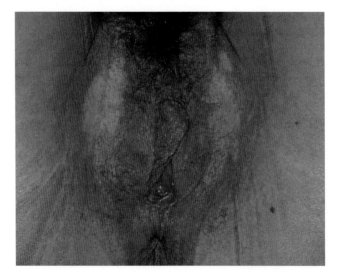

FIGURE 12.3.2   Vitiligo.

Epidemiology: It affects 0.5%–2% of the world's population. It mostly occurs at a young age (20 years of age on average). Vulvar involvement is frequent.

Clinical course: It is a benign disorder with a chronic relapsing course.

Diagnosis: It is clinical. Wood's lamp examination may enhance unnoticed lesions. Biopsy should be reserved to selected cases for ruling out other hypopigmentary disorders.

Differential diagnosis: Postinflammatory hypopigmentation, lichen sclerosus, and piebaldism.

Therapy: Treatment includes topical or systemic corticosteroids and topical calcineurin inhibitors; phototherapy has no role in the management of genital vitiligo. With the involvement of the vulvar area alone, no treatment is recommended other than reassurance.

Bibliography

Kim DY, Lee J, Oh SH, Hann SK, Shin YJ. Impact of genital involvement on the sexual lives of vitiligo patients. *J Dermatol* 2013;40:1065–7.

Patel NS, Paghdal KV, Cohen GF. Advanced treatment modalities for vitiligo. *Dermatol Surg* 2012;38:381–91.

Picardo M. Vitiligo: New insights. *Br J Dermatol* 2012;166:472–3.

Speeckaert R, van Geel N. Distribution patterns in generalized vitiligo. *J Eur Acad Dermatol Venereol* 2014;28:755–62.

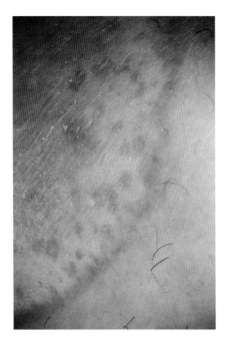

FIGURE 12.3.3   Postinflammatory hypopigmentation following a burn.

12.3.2 Postinflammatory Hypopigmentation

Clinical aspect: The skin color may be lightened (hypopigmented) or completely white (depigmented). The original shape of the eruption is followed (Figure 12.3.3).

Definition: Hypochromic patches with partial loss of epidermal melanin content following a local inflammatory reaction.

Etiology: Temporary or permanent melanocyte damage following any injury causing skin inflammation. Different extrinsic (e.g., burns and ionizing irradiation) or intrinsic (e.g., discoid lupus erythematosus and psoriasis) causes may be pathogenetically involved.

Epidemiology: It is relatively common.

Clinical course: The lesions may be transient or persist indefinitely.

Diagnosis: It is clinical, based on the physical examination and, if necessary, histopathology to rule out other conditions.

Differential diagnosis: Vitiligo and lichen sclerosus.

Therapy: Treatment is not necessary.

Bibliography

Trager JD. What's your diagnosis? Loss of vulvar pigmentation in a two-year-old girl. *J Pediatr Adolesc Gynecol* 2005;18:121–4.

13

Pruritus

Giuseppe Micali, Anna Elisa Verzì, and Francesco Lacarrubba

13.1 Pruritus with or without Excoriations/Fissures

13.1.1 Scabies

Clinical aspect: It is characterized by stubborn itching, which is particularly intense at night, scratch marks and the presence of pathognomonic intraepidermal burrows (cunicula) created by the moving female mite, which appear as serpiginous, grayish, thread-like superficial elevations that are from 2 to 10 mm long. Common sites of infestation include flexor aspects of the wrists, interdigital web spaces of the hands, dorsal feet, axillae, elbows, waist, buttocks, and genitalia. Clinical findings also include small papules, vesicles, and reddish nodules, which correspond to lesions healing with development of an inflammatory granulomatous reaction and are especially common on the male genitalia (nodular scabies) (Figure 13.1.1).

Definition: Scabies is a highly contagious cutaneous ectoparasitosis.

Etiology: It is caused by the mite *Sarcoptes scabiei hominis.* Mites are attracted to the warmth and smell of humans. Pregnant female mites dig burrows into the stratum corneum of the epidermis, creating small, threadlike tunnels (cunicula) and laying eggs at their end. Eggs hatch after 3–4 days and new mites reach adulthood in 15–18 days. Contamination may occur by either direct (notably during sexual intercourse) or indirect contact (clothing and bedding). The mite can survive in the environment for 24–36 hours. Scabies is classified as a sexually transmitted disease.

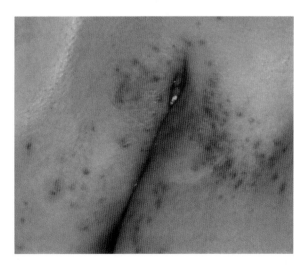

FIGURE 13.1.1   Intensely pruritic erythematous scattered papules: scabies.

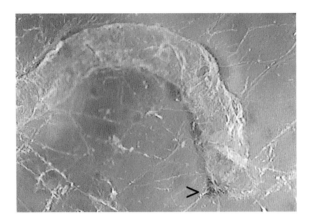

FIGURE 13.1.2 Dermoscopy of scabies: presence of the mite (arrowhead) at the end of a burrow, with a characteristic jet-plane or hang-glider appearance.

Epidemiology: Scabies is a very common disorder. Approximately 300 million cases are reported worldwide each year. It may affect individuals of all ages, races, and socioeconomic classes. In industrialized countries, scabies epidemics occur primarily in institutional settings, such as prisons, and in long-term care facilities, including hospitals and nursing homes.

Clinical course: With proper diagnosis and treatment, the prognosis in otherwise healthy individuals with classic scabies is excellent. If not treated, its course may become chronic and complicated by bacterial superinfections. In debilitated or immunosuppressed patients, the infestation may evolve into a generalized hyperkeratotic and crusty dermatosis, mainly involving the hands and feet, named Norwegian scabies.

Diagnosis: The diagnosis of scabies can often be easily made clinically in patients with a pruritic rash and characteristic linear burrows. It is confirmed by light microscopic identification of mites, larvae, ova, or scybala (feces) in the scales obtained by skin scraping. Dermoscopy, showing the mite with the typical "jet with contrail" aspect at one end of the burrow at low magnifications, or the mite (Figure 13.1.2), its eggs, or feces at higher magnifications, is also an extremely useful noninvasive diagnostic tool.

Differential diagnosis: Misdiagnosis is common and other skin disorders, particularly those causing itching, should be considered, including atopic dermatitis, dermatophytosis, contact dermatitis, Dühring disease, bullous pemphigoid, and psoriasis.

Therapy: Treatment includes topical scabicidal agents (e.g., permethrin, benzyl benzoate, crotamiton, malathion, and lindane), as well as an appropriate antimicrobial agent if a secondary infection has developed. Other treatments include oral ivermectin. Antihistamines may be used to control itching, which may persist for a few weeks after healing. Proper treatment of clothes and bedclothes is essential. Treatment must involve the entire household or community to prevent reinfestation.

Bibliography

Bakos L, Reusch MC, D'Elia P, Aquino V, Bakos RM. Crusted scabies of the vulva. *J Eur Acad Dermatol Venereol* 2007;21:682–4.

Fischer G, Rogers M. Vulvar disease in children: A clinical audit of 130 cases. *Pediatr Dermatol* 2000;17:1–6.

Micali G, Lacarrubba F, Massimino D, Schwartz RA. Dermatoscopy: Alternative uses in daily clinical practice. *J Am Acad Dermatol* 2011;64:1135–46.

Moreland AA. Vulvar manifestations of sexually transmitted diseases. *Semin Dermatol* 1994;13:262–8.

13.1.2 Phthiriasis

Clinical aspect: Small, red, primary papules may be found, but secondary changes from scratching with some serous crusts are usually more obvious. Careful inspection of the genital skin reveals bluish spots, known as maculae caeruleae, secondary to insect bites, which enable the detection of the 1–2-mm, small, tan, or brown lice (Figures 13.1.3 and 13.1.4) and of their whitish, rounded, and elongated nits (eggs) firmly attached to the pubic hair shafts. Pruritus is intense and bothersome.

Definition: Phthiriasis is a lice infestation of the pubic area that may also extend to other hairy body regions (groin, axilla, eyebrow, and eyelash).

Etiology: Phthirus pubis is the pubic louse, whose bites cause intense itching. It lives on humans and is spread by close physical contact either sexually or by fomites (underwear and bedclothes).

Epidemiology: This is a common ectoparasitosis that is diffused worldwide and affects predominantly young, sexually active individuals.

Clinical course: With time, the infestation can extend to other hairy body areas, such as the axillae and eyelashes.

Diagnosis: It is clinical. The louse can be identified *ex vivo* under a microscope. Videodermatoscopy enables detailed *in vivo* identification of both mites and nits (Figure 13.1.5). Full, viable nits appear as

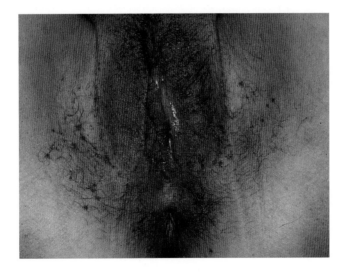

FIGURE 13.1.3 Oozing and reddened vulvar skin from repeated rubbing: phthiriasis.

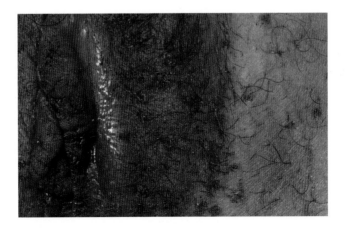

FIGURE 13.1.4 Phthiriasis: at closer inspection brownish lice attached to pubic hairs are evident.

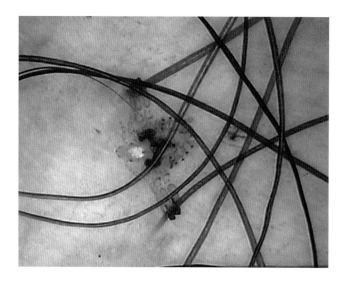

FIGURE 13.1.5   Dermoscopy showing Phthirus pubis grasping two hairs.

opaque structures with a rounded free ending fixed to the hair shaft; empty nits appear as translucent structures with a flat and fissured free ending.

Differential diagnosis: The differential diagnosis may include several other pruritic skin disorders.

Therapy: Effective treatment is based on the use of topical insecticides, such as permethrin 1% cream. Trichotomy may be useful. Treatment of contacts and proper care of underwear and bedclothes is necessary to prevent reinfestation.

Bibliography

Leone PA. Scabies and pediculosis pubis: An update of treatment regimens and general review. *Clin Infect Dis* 2007;44:S153–9.

Micali G, Lacarrubba F, Massimino D, Schwartz RA. Dermatoscopy: Alternative uses in daily clinical practice. *J Am Acad Dermatol* 2011;64:1135–46.

Scott GR, Chosidow O, IUSTI/WHO. European guideline for the management of pediculosis pubis. *Int J STD AIDS* 2011;22:304–5.

Varela JA, Otero L, Espinosa E, Sánchez C, Junquera ML, Vázquez F. Phthirus pubis in a sexually transmitted diseases unit: A study of 14 years. *Sex Transm Dis* 2003;30:292–6.

14

Miscellaneous

Maria Rita Nasca, and Giuseppe Micali

14.1 Mechanical/Obstetric/Surgical Trauma

Clinical aspect: They may cause vulvoperineal tears with bleeding (Figures 14.1.1 and 14.1.2) and genital thrombosis. Perineal tears can be partial, complete, or complicated. Following gynecologic surgery, the patient may report significant hematoma formation and scarring.

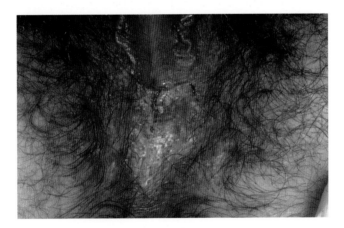

FIGURE 14.1.1   Tear from mechanical trauma.

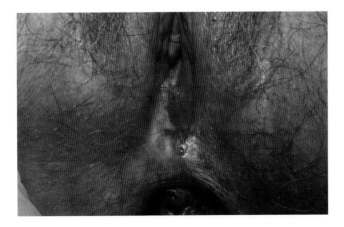

FIGURE 14.1.2   Injury from mechanical trauma.

Definition: They are disorders caused by physical injuries that can involve the vulvar area.

Etiology: They may be due to a precipitous delivery or an overweight newborn. Gynecological surgery is also a possible cause, especially extensive surgery needed for hidradenitis suppurativa, squamous cell carcinoma, Paget disease, or melanoma.

Epidemiology: Obstetric traumas are more common than the other types.

Clinical course: The clinical course is related to the extent of the trauma.

Diagnosis: Clinical history and clinical features are sufficient for diagnosis.

Differential diagnosis: Sexual abuse.

Therapy: Vulvectomy may be considered for some of these patients.

Bibliography

Habek D, Kulas T. Nonobstetrics vulvovaginal injuries: Mechanism and outcome. *Arch Gynecol Obstet* 2007;275:93–7.

Merritt DF. Genital trauma in prepubertal girls and adolescents. *Curr Opin Obstet Gynecol* 2011;23:307–14.

Perkins JD, Morris PF. Traumatic vulvar hematoma masquerading as a Bartholin duct cyst in a postmenopausal woman. *J Miss State Med Assoc* 2013;54:8–10.

Price J. Injuries in prepubertal and pubertal girls. *Best Pract Res Clin Obstet Gynaecol* 2013;27:131–9.

White C. Genital injuries in adults. *Best Pract Res Clin Obstet Gynaecol* 2013;27:113–30.

14.2 Congenital Malformations

14.2.1 Female/Male Pseudohermaphroditism/Disorders of Gonadal Differentiation

Clinical aspect: It depends on the genotype. The patient may have development of both of the genitalia, pseudohermaphroditism, or other possible permutations and combinations of features. In female pseudohermaphroditism, an enlarged phallus, alone or associated with some degree of labioscrotal fusion, is usually observed (Figure 14.2.1), whereas underdevelopment of male genitalia characterizes male pseudohermaphroditism. In gonadal dysgenesis, a normal female phenotype may be present at birth, but pubertal development fails.

Definition: They are congenital abnormalities that affect the external genital organs.

Etiology: Female pseudohermaphroditism is usually caused by a recessive congenital enzymatic defect of adrenal steroid biosynthesis. These patients present a 46 XX genotype with normal ovaries. The most common enzymatic defect is that of the 21-hydroxylase, which causes an overproduction of androgens and an underproduction of cortisol with consequent virilization. Male pseudohermaphroditism may be the result of a lack of gonadotropin, an enzyme defect in testosterone biosynthesis or a defect in androgen-dependent target tissue responses. Disorders of gonadal differentiation may be related to a different number or structure of X and Y chromosomes or to a male-specific transplant antigen (H-Y antigen) that interacts with the Y chromosome to induce testicular differentiation. They can occur in several chromosomal abnormalities, with one of the most common being Turner's syndrome (45X) or Turner's mosaicism (45X/46XX). True hermaphroditism is also possible, with external and internal genital development.

Epidemiology: Developmental abnormalities of the female genital tract are rare. Female pseudohermaphroditism accounts for 80% of ambiguous genitalia, whereas male pseudohermaphroditism occurs in approximately 15% of cases.

Clinical course: It is uneventful.

Diagnosis: It is clinical, but requires hormonal and genetic investigations.

Differential diagnosis: Other congenital malformations must be ruled out.

Therapy: Pediatric patients with ambiguous genitalia must be immediately assessed.

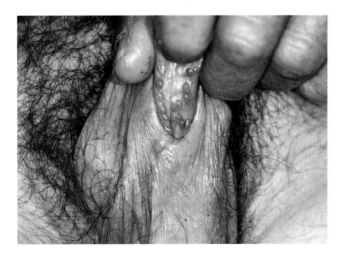

FIGURE 14.2.1   Pseudohermaphroditism.

Bibliography

Al-Maghribi H. Congenital adrenal hyperplasia: Problems with developmental anomalies of the external genitalia and sex assignment. *Saudi J Kidney Dis Transpl* 2007;18:405–13.

Hughes IA, Nihoul-Fékété C, Thomas B, Cohen-Kettenis PT. Consequences of the ESPE/LWPES guidelines
for diagnosis and treatment of disorders of sex development. *Best Pract Res Clin Endocrinol Metab*
2007;21:351–65.

Yankovic F, Cherian A, Steven L, Mathur A, Cuckow P. Current practice in feminizing surgery for congenital
adrenal hyperplasia; a specialist survey. *J Pediatr Urol* 2013;9:1103–7.

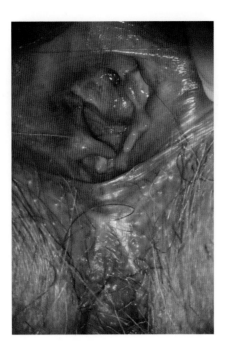

FIGURE 14.2.2 Hymenal abnormality.

14.2.2 Hymenal Abnormalities

Clinical aspect: In these abnormalities, the hymen is completely or partially intact (Figure 14.2.2). The vagina is distended and may be large and sausage-shaped. The patient may present with amenorrhea associated with lower abdominal discomfort.

Definition: The hymen is a thin membrane of connective tissue that surrounds or partially covers the external vaginal opening. Different patterns may occur, including several microperforations (cribriform/fenestrated hymen) or a nonexistent hymenal opening (imperforate hymen).

Etiology: They are congenital and involve the failure of complete or uniform embryonic canalization. Partial canalization may be caused by recurrent vaginal infection in the prepubertal years as a result of trapped secretions, urine, and bacteria.

Epidemiology: These abnormalities are uncommon.

Clinical course: The condition is usually noticed cyclically for 1–3 months or more with severe cyclical lower abdominal pain.

Diagnosis: It is clinical, including history of the patient, physical examination and, occasionally, ultrasound.

Differential diagnosis: Labial adhesions.

Therapy: For an imperforate hymen, a surgical hymenotomy is recommended.

Bibliography

Anthuber S, Strauss A, Anthuber C, Hepp H. Abnormalities of external and internal genitalia. *Gynakol Geburtshilfliche Rundsch* 2003;43:136–45.

Basaran M, Usal D, Aydemir C. Hymen sparing surgery for imperforate hymen: Case reports and review of literature. *J Pediatr Adolesc Gynecol* 2009;22:e61–4.

Kimberley N, Hutson JM, Southwell BR, Grover SR. Vaginal agenesis, the hymen, and associated anomalies. *J Pediatr Adolesc Gynecol* 2012;25:54–8.

Lankford JC, Mancuso P, Appel R. Congenital reproductive abnormalities. *J Midwifery Womens Health* 2013;58:546–551.

Index

A

Abuse, 129, 172, 190
Acantholytic dyskeratosis, 55
Acanthosis nigricans, 180; *see also* Pigmentary
    changes 83, 169
ACD, *see* Allergic CD (ACD)
Acne inversa, *see* Hidradenitis suppurativa
Acquired junctional melanocytic nevus, 177
Acrochordon, 150–151; *see also* Nodules 94, 119, 124
Acrodermatitis enteropathica, 5, 16, 18, 24, 27, 29, 31
Acute candidiasis, 17, 18
Acute contact dermatitis, 24
Acute fixed drug eruption, 9–10
Acute napkin dermatitis, 23
AIDS, 76, 109, 110; *see also* HIV
Allergic CD (ACD), 23, 51
Amicrobic pustulosis of the folds, 69, 70
Angioedema, 35; *see also* 20, 38
Angiofibroma, 154; *see also* Nodules
Angiokeratoma, 84–86; *see also* 107, 110, 171, 172
Angiokeratoma of Mibelli, 86
Angiosarcoma, 107, 110
Anogenital warts, 117–119; *see also* 76, 78, 86, 90, 94,
    112, 116, 120, 124, 125
Aphthosis, 165–166; *see also* Ulcers 42, 46
Aspergillosis, 76
Atopic dermatitis, 30–31; *see also* 5, 8, 16, 18, 24, 27, 29,
    33, 52, 57, 137, 140, 186

B

Bacillary angiomatosis, 107, 110
Bacterial infections, 5, 8, 12, 13, 15, 18, 21, 27, 31,
    50, 52, 61, 62, 65, 73, 83, 132, 133, 135, 140,
    167, 169
Bartholin's glands, 1–3, 21
Basal cell carcinoma, 124; *see also* 76, 81, 88, 90, 94,
    143, 156, 175, 177
BD, *see* Behçet disease (BD)
Behçet disease (BD), 165–166; *see also* Ulcers 42, 99
Benign familial pemphigus, *see* Hailey–Hailey disease
Benign vulvar melanosis, 174, 175; *see also* Pigmentary
    changes 173
Blisters, *see* Vesicles and Bullae
Bowenoid papulosis, 89–90; *see also* 88, 119, 143
Bowen's disease, 143; *see also* Plaques 90
Bruise, 171–172; *see also* Pigmentary changes 128
Bullous pemphigoid, 58–59; *see also* 9, 54, 58, 63, 65,
    105, 123, 186
Buschke-Loewenstein tumor, 119

C

Candidiasis, 17–19, 67, 68; *see also* 5, 8, 12, 13, 15, 16,
    21, 24, 27, 29, 31, 33, 52, 70, 132, 133, 135,
    137, 140
Cayenne pepper spotting, 131
CD, *see* Contact dermatitis (CD); Crohn's disease (CD)
Cellulitis, 20; *see also* 35, 38, 48
Cervical endometriosis, 96
Cervical trichomoniasis, 11–12
Chancre, *see* Primary syphilis
Chancroid, 161–162; *see also* 39, 42, 46, 69, 99, 147,
    164, 166
Chickenpox, 49–50; *see also* 48
Chlamydial infections, 12, 21, 39, 96
Chronic candidiasis, 19
Cicatricial pemphigoid, 54, 59, 61, 65, 105, 123, 129
Clear cell acanthoma, 94, 124
Clitoris, 2
Coccidioidomycosis, 76, 138, 167
Condyloma, 21, 117–119; *see also* Anogenital warts
Condylomata lata, *see* Secondary syphilis
Congenital dermal melanocytic nevus, 94
Congenital dystrophic epidermolysis bullosa, 65
Congenital junctional melanocytic nevus, 178
Congenital malformations, 191
Contact dermatitis (CD), 23–24, 28–29, 51–52; *see also*
    5, 8, 16, 18, 20, 27, 31, 33, 35, 38, 48, 135, 137,
    138, 140, 142, 169, 186
Crohn's disease (CD), 41–42; *see also* 39, 69, 73, 166
Cryptococcosis, 76, 167
Cysts, 157
    epidermal inclusion cyst, 159–160
    vestibular mucous cyst, 157–158

D

Darier disease, 83; *see also* 5, 8, 16, 18, 24, 27, 29, 113
Dermal melanocytic nevus, 93–95
Dermatitis herpetiformis, *see* Dühring disease
Dermatofibroma, 94, 124
Dermatome, 47
Dermatophytosis, 25–27; *see also* 5, 8, 16, 18, 24, 29, 31,
    33, 61, 70, 105, 135, 137, 140, 169, 186
Dermoscopy of
    acquired dermal melanocytic nevus, 94
    anogenital warts, 119
    inverse psoriasis, 8
    junctional melanocytic nevus, 178
    lichen planus, 105
    molluscum contagiosum, 76